Praise for Gut Guide 101

"This is truly a practical guide to good digestive health. I found the recommendations to be research based and uncomplicated. The book is a great tool for those of us who want to feel better but need to make changes in small steps."

- Brooke Stratton, Overland Park, KS

Special Ed Administrator

"Hahn's style is genuine and her enthusiasm is infectious."

- Stephanie Stalmah, Valparaiso, IN

Program Director

"I was having acid reflux and a lot of gas. That's when Mari Hahn came out with her 21-Day Plan for Better Digestion and Increased Energy. I decided to give it a try and honestly, I did not expect it to help me as much as it did. Almost immediately, I was feeling better and I forgot that I ever had acid reflux. Her approach is very simple and direct. It is all laid out in easy to understand and easy to follow terms. I highly recommend it. This is a book I will use with my own health coaching clients and is a great giveaway for other health coaches to use with their clients, too."

- Patty Swiatly, Chicago, IL
Massage Therapist, Health Coach

"The 21-Day Plan was super easy to understand and implement."

- Troy Ford, Beverly Shores, IN

Personal Trainer, Owner of Troybuilt Fitness

"I didn't think I had any issues with my digestion but I really felt better after trying the 21-Day Plan. I love the way this book is so positive and how it suggests you add onto your routine instead of taking away foods like other 'diets.'"

> *- Amanda Freymann, Beverly Shores, IN*
> *Publications Consultant*

"I felt like you wrote this book just for me."

> *- Dawn Sciarra, Valparaiso, IN*
> *Hair Stylist*

"This is more of a healthy lifestyle book than a 'diet' book. We frequently hear that fats, sweets, and red meat are bad for us. Hahn has gone a few steps further and explained the specifics about how vegetables, fruits, water, good quality proteins, and other healthy, whole foods nourish our bodies!"

> *- Patti Kirk, Valparaiso, IN*
>
> *Stay-at-home Mom*

"I absolutely loved your book. It's a complete guide and awesome tool!! Very easy 'to digest.'"

> *- Elena Petcu, Constanta, Romania*
>
> *Health Coach*

"It was one of the easiest plans to follow. I love the fact that it encourages adding things in instead of taking things out."

> *- Ellen Hundt, Beverly Shores, IN*

"Pretty straightforward and easy."

> *- Karla Gray, St. Louis, MO*

GUT GUIDE 101: THREE WEEKS TO BETTER DIGESTION AND INCREASED ENERGY

Mari J Hahn

Published by Alive and Well

ISBN: 0990744701

ISBN-13: 978-0-9907447-0-2

Table of Contents

Introduction

America is facing a health crisis. Some may call it an obesity crisis while others use the term "diabesity." We know we have a growing epidemic of health related issues due to our ever-increasing weight. We worry about the escalating rates of heart disease and cancer. We are seeing accelerating rates of many preventable diseases in our children. Quite simply, our collective health is in jeopardy. But it goes even deeper than that. For millions of people, every day is a physical struggle. *We just don't feel good.* We have access to an array of thousands of foods, top scientists and advanced medicine and yet our most basic measure of health – how we feel each day – is failing.

Our bodies are miraculous, intricate organisms with hundreds of systems to keep everything working. For many health issues, our body "knows" how to get back in balance, without us even giving it a thought. Yet, somehow, many of us are not in balance at all. So, what gives? The truth is, much of the problem leads back to our digestive system. Our digestion is our "intake system" allowing us to eat and drink whatever we want. The digestive system then assimilates it all throughout our bodies, getting the nutrients to all the cells that need them, getting rid of what is not needed through the bowels and fighting off invaders that try to take over. However, when we are constipated, when we have diarrhea or our gut bacteria is damaged, this amazing system comes to a screeching halt. We do not get the nutrients we need. We feel fatigued every day. We are not operating at our best. We can barely get through the day. We don't sleep well at night. Our digestive system cannot get rid of the toxins and waste products. We are more susceptible to disease and illness. We are literally clogged with toxins and waste. Our bodies are crying for help. Yet, many of us are out of touch with the signals.

What we see on TV and what we read in the mainstream media only confuses us further. We receive many conflicting messages and thousands of well-crafted advertisements (which are designed to make the company money, not make us healthy) telling us what to eat and drink. "Coffee is bad for you" "Coffee is good for you" "Fat is good for you" "Fat is bad for you" "Carbs are bad for you" "Carbs are good for you" "Meat is good for you" "Meat is bad for you" "A glass of wine is bad for you" "A glass of wine is good for you" "Chocolate is good for you" "Chocolate is bad for you."

It's so hard to make any sense of it all. If we were trying to make decisions about what to eat today based on the media, our diets would do a 180 every week!

A good and reliable way to make sense of it does exist. You have one ultimate authority on what your body needs. And that is......*your body*! Each of us has our own unique set of systems, our own unique DNA, our own unique set of gut bacteria. All of those things influence what each person needs to thrive. It seems like a secret code. But it's not secret at all if you know how to listen to your body.

We are going to learn to decipher the code. We are going to learn how to become more conscious of what our bodies are telling us. This book will help you become a detective and a scientist – a super sleuth of your own digestive system. I want to introduce you to your "Inner Doctor." Let's call him/her I.D. Your I.D. is going to ask a lot of questions and look for symptoms and maybe even explore some health issues you thought were just something you were going to have to live with for the rest of your life. Chapter by chapter, you will decipher the messages your body is sending and learn how to take action. This makes it sound complicated. Really, it's not. I just ask that you open yourself to new ways of looking at your health.

We do have some obstacles to get around, though. Our modern western diets have blurred the signals and symptoms for our Inner Doctor. If you ask your I.D. what your body is hungry for and the answer you get is Chocolate Salted Caramel Cupcake, then you know you have some extra layers of signals to decipher. You may really *be* hungry for that cupcake. It has the salt and sugar and fat that your taste buds and your brain (and maybe even your gut bacteria) crave. But on some level you know that the cupcake will not provide the nutrients, vitamins and minerals that will help your body function at its best and thrive. Plus you may get a bellyache and feel sluggish after eating the cupcake. We need to gain a better understanding of our cravings, where they come from, and how to tame them. For many of us, we need to get our systems (especially our digestive system, or gut) in better working order. Don't worry. This book will lead you step by step to do just that.

Another obstacle is the actual food that we consume. Much of our food these days is highly processed and can contain harmful ingredients that throw off or damage our digestive systems. This book provides the information needed to better understand the hidden dangers in our food. We will start with small changes. You may be surprised to find out that often a few simple changes to your diet, some extra water, and two gut-friendly supplements can make a big difference in your digestion. Once you begin to feel better, you may want to take things to the next level, and you will have the information to do that.

The book is divided into two sections. Part One will help you understand the digestive system better and learn about different influences on digestion. Part Two consists of many helpful tools to make simple changes over the course of three weeks and beyond. Throughout the book, you will see many references marked in (parentheses such as this) which refer to an article or research study. At the end of the book you will find the complete list of referenced articles to locate more information on a particular study or topic. Check out the recommended books, websites, apps and movies for easy ways to further your education. Perhaps, you may want to share these with a friend or family member. Chapter 7 gives detailed instructions and action steps to improve your own digestion. Chapter 8 details how to listen to your body and deconstruct the signals it is sending. Chapter 9 will help you develop a daily plan for fitting in some exercise that will fit *your* lifestyle. Of course, stress negatively affects our digestion as well as our energy level. Chapter 10 will address that with plenty of tools to help you reduce the harmful effects of stress. Chapter 11 provides delicious, gut-friendly recipes for every meal of the day plus delicious snacks and desserts. First things first – read this book. After reading the book, prepare to implement the simple 21-Day Plan for Better Digestion and Increased Energy. Before you begin, fill out the symptom chart on page 66. Then decide which day you wish to begin your 21-Day Plan and purchase the needed supplies. The handy shopping list tells you exactly what to buy. The action steps are phased in over three weeks to make it easier to fit into your daily schedule.

Keep in mind, many excellent books have already been written on digestion and improving your gut health. I have studied many of them and you may have, too. They contain great information;

however, I find most of the advice is very challenging and compli-cated to follow. Many involve giving up major food groups completely and quitting your favorite foods "cold turkey." Many involve preparing all of your food at home, even though most of us regularly eat at restaurants or eat "on the go." In short, they involve big changes to your daily schedule and lifestyle. *Making big, sweeping changes to your diet is not required to start enjoying better digestion and increased energy.* These dramatic changes to your diet and lifestyle, while they may be helpful for your digestion, are very difficult for many people to follow and therefore, the success rate is low. I want you to be successful. I want you to have better digestion and increased energy. *Gut Guide 101* is intended for people who are busy – people who may not have the time or motivation or money to make *major* changes. Maybe you have very little experience making changes to your diet, or maybe you have tried plans in the past but were not successful due to the difficulty level of the plan. *Gut Guide 101* is a moderate approach – based on the idea that small changes can make a big difference.

With *this* plan, in a few short weeks your digestion will be in better working order and you will be feeling better. You will be sleeping more soundly. You will be eliminating toxins more efficiently. You will have more energy to do the things you love to do each day. If you want to take it a step or two further, visit www.gutguide101.com for further workshops and online webinars.

You are going to start to think of your digestive system (your gut) in a whole new way. And you are going to feel a whole lot better in the process!

The Main Concepts of the 21-Day Plan for Better Digestion and Increased Energy:

- More water every day
- Meet your new breakfast smoothie
- More fiber and nutrients every day in the form of whole fruit and green veggies
- Start the day with a glass of water with lemon juice to "set the stage" for good digestion all day – alkalinizes the body
- Add in fermented foods
- Green tea everyday – for antioxidants and anti-inflammatory properties
- Probiotic cultures – through yogurt and probiotic supplement
- Magnesium citrate at bedtime to calm the body for good sleep and good digestion
- Move your body everyday

PART ONE
1| Inspiration to Change

"Sometimes it's the smallest decisions that can change your life."
-Keri Russell

My Uncle Ray has a beer belly. He pats it affectionately and says, "It's the only thing I own that's paid for!" We laugh at the funny joke. I am struck by this thought of ownership. He owns that? Like you own a car? OK. Maybe not like that. When your car breaks down you can buy a new part and have it installed. In fact, you can trade in the whole car for a brand new one when it stops running. The more I thought about it, I began to realize, Uncle Ray was wrong – at least in part. He's right about the ownership, but it's not paid for. He's paying for it now.

Ray has high blood pressure, fatigue, acid reflux and weakening muscles. He's also what is called "pre-diabetic." These are the costs of "owning" that gut. He's often been told to quit eating fried foods, to quit this and to quit that. He does none of those things for more than a few days. He's tried and he couldn't. And neither could I. (The failure eats away at self-esteem, doesn't it)? Then, since I love my Uncle Ray, it occurred to me that maybe taking things away from him wasn't the best way to begin. Maybe we could begin by adding in a few things. More on that later....

So, you may be asking yourself how a massage therapist gets involved in studying the gut. In the early 1990's I went to massage school – Jay Scherer's Academy of Natural Healing – in beautiful Santa Fe, New Mexico. It was an amazing education in a beautiful location. I learned a lot about massage therapy, but also, I learned to look at the body as a whole organism. The body has multiple amazing systems to keep itself in balance. The body *wants* to be in balance. Sometimes we give our doctor or the medical community full credit for healing what is wrong with us, but that's simply not true. People's bodies have been healing themselves for a lot longer than we have had western medicine! Think about it – if you break your arm, you probably go to the emergency room and get an x-ray. They confirm, "Yes, it is broken." The doctor puts on a cast and gives you something for the pain. They might even do surgery. And in a few weeks they remove the cast and, voila. Your arm is not broken anymore! Did the people at the E.R. do that? Or the cast? No. Your body healed itself. It is a miraculous process that goes on in the body whereby cells regenerate and repair, crowding out and eventually getting rid of the damaged cells. The doctors and the cast are certainly helpful. If it were not for them, the arm bone might not have healed in a straight line causing pain in the future or decreased function. But even after all of that, it is the processes that go on inside your body at the cellular level that actually do the healing.

Imagine something even more basic – a paper cut. Yesterday I got a paper cut from my son's schoolwork. It hurt like heck for a few minutes, even bled a little. Then that cellular regeneration and repair process began without my even giving it a thought. Today, I am looking at my finger. It doesn't hurt anymore. It certainly is not bleeding. There is a tiny bit of redness, but for the most part the little cut is almost completely healed in less than 24 hours. So, not only does our body have a whole host of mechanisms for healing itself and bringing itself back into balance, day after day, year after year, but also it does all this in a very short amount of time. Why is this? Because, the longer things are out of balance, the harder it is for the body to get things *back* into balance. The body acts quickly. If too many things are out of balance for long periods of time, well, the short answer is – you can die. All of the body's mechanisms exist for one simple reason – for your survival!

Now the body has all these great systems in place. But that doesn't mean it can do *everything* all by itself. It needs some basic raw ingredients to work with. It needs water for basic cell function. It needs calories for energy. But not just any calories – it needs nourishing vitamins, minerals and enzymes, phytochemicals and other nutrients that allow the cells in different parts of our bodies to fully function. We get these through a variety of fruits, vegetables, fats, seeds, nuts, grains, beans and animal products. These are the food components that have been shown to be crucial to our healthy cell function throughout our whole system. We also need clean air to breathe. This provides the vital oxygen for our cells. These cell functions are occurring all over our body, 24/7 – through muscle movement, neurological function, organ function, brain function and, well, you get the idea.

Back to my story. After massage school, I went on to work as a massage therapist for 20 years. I worked on many clients who taught me how incredible the human body is! I saw many people heal from all kinds of pain, injuries and ailments. I also saw many people struggle. Some struggled with multiple health problems and had trouble healing and getting back into balance. I struggled with my own weight and health issues during that time. Throughout that same 20-year time frame, the disease trends in the U.S., and many other developed countries, have shown accelerated rates of many preventable diseases. We, as a society, are saddled with high rates of obesity, heart disease, cancer, Type 2 diabetes, and stroke. Many kids are not healthy. Many adults are not healthy. And why is that? Why now?

Mountains of new research, my own experience as well as careful firsthand observations over many years as a wellness practitioner, have resulted in narrowing down the root of the problem. It's in Uncle Ray! OK, it's in me, too and you, as well, but it's fun to point the finger elsewhere, isn't it? Much of the problem starts in our digestive system – we'll call it our gut. It's in our microbiome. (Sounds like a mini-series by Stephen King, doesn't it?) Well, we all have one. Here's what the dictionary says about it: *"Microbiome, Noun. The totality of microorganisms and their collective genetic material present in or on the human body, or in another environment."* (Random House Dictionary 2014) How about that? You have microorganisms *in your body*. They live *in your gut*. Your gut is an environment! That makes you an environmentalist of your own ecosystem. Hey, you own it, remember? This book will give you a plan for its care and feeding.

Back to Uncle Ray. The idea of ownership stuck with me and motivated me through the years. Do you know the pride and satisfaction of making something, writing something, cooking something, fixing something, or creating something? It's a special satisfaction because you did it yourself, with your own hands. And it is real – not abstract. It is much better than the false sense of ownership you get when you simply buy something. This digestive system, or gut – you own it. You can do something with it, and for it. You can create a life with more energy, where you wake up in the morning feeling great. You can boost your immunity and even increase your life expectancy!

Do you have trouble losing weight? Do you suffer with arthritis, joint pain, low energy, constipation, diarrhea, nausea, acid reflux

(GERD), allergies, skin problems, or depression? Do you crave sugar, alcohol, cigarettes or caffeine? Wouldn't it be wonderful to be free of those issues? These are clearly obstacles to good health, to good energy, to a positive outlook on life and to nights of sound sleep. And they are all closely linked to your digestive system. Your immune system is also closely intertwined with digestive health. Over 70% of our immune system lives in the gut (Vighi 2008). If you catch every cold and flu bug going around, that is a sign that your gut environment is not functioning at its best. Daily fatigue and brain fog can also be traced back to poor digestive health. These discomforts are all warning signals. "Help!" is the message our gut is sending us. "Send some help!" Get your gut in better working order and in a surprisingly short time (remember, the body heals fast, when given half a chance) you will start to feel much better.

Picture a coral reef in all its brilliance, its fiery spectrums, coral and living sea plants. It is a living thing. Everything works together in an eco-system: the dancing plants – all the myriad forms of marine life. It is wondrously complex and beautiful to behold. We must respect it if it is to thrive. This is also how your digestive system is made to work, as an open and complex system. The bacteria in your gut are in a lovely place. They are all working together to keep you healthy and balanced. Vital nutrients are easily assimilated into your bloodstream giving you energy and life force. You are being protected as well. The system, running smoothly and efficiently, makes sure that toxins are removed daily. It's amazing and it, too, needs care and respect. Let's take a closer look at it.

Your digestive system is an open tube through your body from your mouth to your anus. This is how your body takes in things from the outside world. Everything that you put in your mouth, from a glass of water, to that fast food meal, to that salad, to your meds, to your 3 daily glasses of wine – simply put – goes into your digestive tract where your gut "decides" what to do with it. It has four main options: 1: It decides it recognizes and can use the substance, and those nutrients or liquids get absorbed into the body to help in your daily activity. 2: It decides it cannot use the substance and then passes it through to be discarded through your stool. 3: It cannot recognize the substance or we ate too much of it which puts added stress on the body. But, never fear! The body is amazing and has a plan for what to do with the excess – storing the unrecognized or excess substance as fat, so it can attend to more important work and never give it another thought. 4: The fourth thing that can, and does, happen, is that the consumed substance actually damages the gut lining itself – it could be a toxin or food that your body cannot digest, or an antibiotic, for example – which causes damage on its way through the tubular system. This is just one reason why you need to keep things moving at a decent pace – you don't want the toxic stuff to be in there, lingering, for any more time than necessary.

As you can see, it's a pretty amazing system. Every day each of our guts is trying its best to take whatever we put in our mouths and use it to keep all of our systems running smoothly. When we are not feeling our best or we are suffering with some of those daily pains and ailments that many people will tell you are just signs of getting older, it's time to take a closer look. Your gut wants you to make some changes. We owe it to ourselves to do just that. We are about to learn simple changes we can make. We must pay attention. Because you own your gut. Just like Uncle Ray.

2| Digestive Woes

The Signals

Your body asks for the help it needs from you. You may not recognize the request. A friend of mine has been telling me for a long time about her six-year-old son's poor health. She took him to many doctors with few results. Finally, recently, she tested him for celiac disease – an autoimmune reaction to eating gluten. He does not have celiac disease; however, the tests showed he is highly sensitive to gluten. As a responsible mom, she is scratching her head and saying, "How can that be? He had no symptoms." Well, he absolutely *did* have symptoms. They just weren't the ones she was looking for. She thought a food allergy would present itself as itching or sneezing. But our bodies send a wide range of different signals. He didn't feel good. He didn't want to get out of bed in the morning. He had a low energy level. He got sick often. These symptoms are not normal for a six-year-old. She thought these were signs of him being stubborn or lazy. She didn't realize that they were his body sending cries for help because he had a food sensitivity. Most types of discomfort, pain or fatigue are messages from our body – "This is not working for me. Please make a change."

I live in the Chicago area. People are crazy about their deep-dish pizza here. You could get a heated discussion going if you ask which deep dish pizza restaurant is the best. I do, on occasion, enjoy some Chicago-style deep-dish pizza. In case you haven't had this pizza before, the crust is formed into a deep pizza pan so that it can hold a deep layer of sauce, toppings and literally pounds of melted cheese. My favorite is the black olive/spinach. But when I eat it, my body sends me a number of signals afterwards that are hard to ignore. I get acid reflux, an overstuffed feeling, stomach gurgling, and later, constipation. These signals are my gut telling me – hey, I cannot process that much cheese and acidic sauce and fat all at one time!

As a nation, our bodies are crying for help. We are dying of preventable diseases in record numbers. Our obesity rate is skyrocketing. In 1996, none of the fifty states had an obesity rate above 20%. Now, in 2014, *every* state has an obesity rate of 21% or higher. The states with the highest obesity rate are up to 35.1% ("Adult Obesity Facts" 2014). In 18 short years we have ballooned into a very overweight nation. The U.S. is second only to Mexico in highest obesity rate ("Obesity Update" 2014). Our bodies are sending SOS signals by the dozens. Yet, many Americans are still driving through McDonald's every day! My kids are 16 and 12 years old. If the increase in Type 2 diabetes diagnosis continues at its current rate, by the time my kids are 40, one third of their peers will have developed Type 2 Diabetes (Fuhrman 2005). That brings with it a host of health problems. We are entering uncharted territory with one third of the population living with Type 2 diabetes for a majority of their lives. Kids' bodies are sending them plenty of signals, but they don't know how to respond. As parents, we need to prioritize getting them some help now to get them on a better path – a path of better digestive health.

The body wants to be in balance. We have many systems in our body – hormonal, adrenal, nervous, digestive, and circulatory – all working 24/7 to keep our bodies in balance. So, how did things go so awry? Why are we in the U.S. worse off than so much of the world? The kids are our canary in the coalmine. Kids are supposed to be healthy and full of life, yet today many kids are having health issues earlier in their lives than ever before. We need to take notice. Why are our kids getting Type 2 diabetes – a disease that used to be associated with the elderly? Why are our kids becoming obese? Fifty or even 30 years ago, kids ate sweets and French fries and junk food. Kids overate. But their bodies eventually told them to stop. They eventually got full and stopped eating. Then an hour later or the next day they felt a little sick. So they naturally ate less – or at least less candy and fries. So why are kids' bodies not telling them to stop eating?

Canary in the coalmine:
Before they had modern gas detection systems, miners would lower a caged canary down into the mine to test the air quality. When they lifted the canary back up, if it was dead, the miners would know the air was not safe to breathe.

It's much more complicated than simply a matter of "calories in, calories out." "Calories in, calories out" refers to the idea that your weight gain or loss is based on simply adding up the number of calories you take in and subtracting the number of calories you expend each day. Rubner invented this "isodynamic law" in 1878. Recent research is showing that the quality and type of food actually does matter over time (Taubes 2012).

And obesity is not simply a lack of willpower to resist overeating, as many believe (Glickman 2012). Our willpower as a society has not changed dramatically in the past twenty years – just our waistlines.

The Perfect Storm

It is a complex problem – a perfect storm. Many internal and external factors that we face every day are affecting our health. Many of these issues have only emerged in the past few decades.

1) Our bodies are starved for nutrients so the body sends signals to eat more food.

2) Everywhere we turn we find an overwhelming availability of junk food and processed food and consumption habits that are ingrained in our culture.

3) The addition of High Fructose Corn Syrup (HFCS) and sugar in its many forms to nearly every prepared food we eat is making us crave even more sugar. This causes an insulin reaction in our bodies that is overwhelming our pancreas, causing imbalance.

4) We are addicted to flavorings, additives and preservatives that are manufactured specifically to hook us on certain foods (Warner 2013). I call this "Capitalism gone wild".

5) "Supersized" and ginormous portions encourage us to eat many times more calories than our bodies need.

6) Many of our meals consist of processed food, packaged food, restaurant meals, fast food, and deep fat fried food that provide plenty of calories but not the nutrients that we need.

7) We've reduced our daily activity level – our 21st century sedentary lifestyles encourage too much time spent sitting in front of a screen (Did you see the movie *Wall-E*?).

8) We have high stress levels: Stress=cortisol=belly fat (pg. 113).

9) Genetically Modified Organisms (GMO), antibiotics, antibacterial hand sanitizers and other toxic substances we put into our bodies interfere with the good gut bacteria in our microbiome.

10) Many people have an imbalance of gut bacteria and a lack of diversity in their microbiome.

11) Chronic inflammation in our bodies causes us to be in a state of constant crisis, putting out fires, so to speak, instead of maintaining a calm state of balance.

12) We know that being born vaginally gives newborn babies a healthy dose of the mother's living microorganisms. Babies born by C-section do not get that same benefit. The CDC reports that in 2012, the C-section rate was 32.8% of births in the U.S.

My son plays a computer game with an interesting feature. You direct your game character to go around attacking other characters just like many other computer games. But his game also has a graphic to let you know when you need to take care of yourself so you don't die. It indicates by a little scale on the sidebar when you need to eat and when you need to sleep and when you need healing. If you don't eat or sleep or get help when the signal gets to the danger level, you die. I love the idea of a signal to tell you how healthy you are. How handy! If only we could have that same signal for our real lives. But, wait – we do. We just ignore the signals. When we reach exhaustion level, we just keep on going. When we have a low level of health, we often do not look at the root causes and try to address the underlying issues. When we are hungry for more nutrients, unfortunately, we often eat heavily processed foods that do not provide the nutrients we need. Over time, ignoring these signals can cause major health problems and yes, even death.

If I asked a room full of people, who wants to drastically change your diet starting tomorrow? How many people do you think would raise their hands?

I can tell you – not many. We are emotionally, physically and psychologically attached to our food on many levels. Yet, largely due to our diets, kids born today are the first generation of Americans whose life expectancy is *less* than their parents ("Obesity Threatens…" 2005). So, we know we need to make a change.

"External Food Disposal System"

Here's an idea: we could all get a new surgically installed "External Food Disposal System" that I have envisioned. It's a switch that is installed on your neck. When you are eating and drinking nourishing foods and beverages that are beneficial to your health, you turn the switch to "ON" so that food goes into your digestive system and gets digested and absorbed. If you are about to eat a food or beverage which does not provide any health benefit and has little nutritional value, you need to remember to turn the switch to "OFF." Then the food gets swallowed, but that is as far as it gets. It gets intercepted and leaves through a hole in your neck and goes into the "External Food Disposal System." You still get to consume the food, enjoying the taste, chewing and swallowing the food, but instead of having it enter your digestive system, it exits your body early, through your neck. The trick is, you need to know when to turn the switch "ON" and "OFF." You need to know which foods are good and helpful to your system and which foods are going to get stored as excess fat, or worse, do damage to your digestive system. That's when you turn the switch to "OFF!"

I know what you are thinking. *That's crazy!*

Of course it is crazy!

Do you know a *real solution?* It doesn't involve some crazy surgery. Where do we start to heal this health crisis of enormous proportions?

Recent research points overwhelmingly to the digestive system.

Digestive Health

Ask yourself, "How do I feel?" The answer can often be a clue to our digestive health.

When our digestive health is at its optimum, we feel creative, energetic, motivated, pain-free, even-tempered. When our digestive health is moderately OK – we might feel "like we are surviving," "getting by," "busy," "stressed." When our digestive health is damaged, then we feel "sick," "in pain," "irritable," "stuck," "exhausted."

When we feel that way we know that change is needed. Can you make changes to heal your gut? Yes, you can! It's not difficult to begin adding in a few foods and supplements over the course of three weeks. You don't have to change everything all at once. By simply improving your digestion, you will be taking a step in a good direction.

3| Gut Bacteria and The Microbiome

"The path to health is paved with good intestines."

-Sherry A. Rogers

The Microbiome

My mom tells a story about her experience in the hospital when she gave birth to me. She wanted to breastfeed. But it wasn't "in style" at the time. It was the 1960's. It was common to give the mother-to-be anesthesia; the doctor delivered the baby and when the woman woke up, the nurse handed her the baby. The dad was out in the waiting room. In my case, my dad tells about watching the All Star baseball game in the waiting room with Uncle Ray while I was born. But I digress. After I was born, the hospital nurses insisted that before my mom fed me, she clean her nipples with an antiseptic to kill any germs before I latched on. I didn't like to latch on. My mom is convinced it was because I didn't like the taste of the antiseptic. (And really, can you blame me?) So the nurses were standing by with a bottle of formula, ready to feed me when the breastfeeding failed. Sad. Do you think breastfeeding babies one hundred or one thousand years ago used antiseptic wipes for their mother's nipples before they latched on? Of course not. They didn't need to. Our bodies have a *natural* antiseptic for our nipples... and everywhere else. This protective layer of bacteria on our skin and in all our body cavities lives in harmony with and is a big part of our immune system. It is called the microbiome (Grice 2011). When it is in balance, it fights off diseases before they even have a chance to enter our individual ecosystem. Our microbiome is keeping the nipples ready for that baby's mouth. We don't need the hospital's antiseptic! As a matter of fact, the living organisms from the mother's skin actually help populate the baby's microbiome. Breast milk itself has living organisms as well as antiseptic properties. This system is especially useful to get the baby's microbiome off to a good start. Do you know where a lot of these bacteria live? We now know it's the gut.

Microbiome refers to the microorganisms in a particular environment including the body or part of the body.

What we have been taught since grade school is wrong – bacteria are not all "bad." They cannot even easily categorized as "good" or "bad." For decades we have been fighting against bacteria, but in fact, we are now realizing that what we thought was "bad" may be working together in this grand scheme that we do not fully understand. The human body is a carefully balanced system that includes 100 trillion microbes (Pollan 2013). These microbes live in relationship with us on our skin, in every body cavity and, it turns out, even inside our entire digestive tract – which technically, is a long tube open to the world.

While bacteria are not easily categorized as all "good" and all "bad," we want to maintain balance and diversity. Certain types are more helpful and certain types are less helpful and a few are downright nasty. We want to maintain a ratio so that the more helpful bacteria outnumber and crowd out the nasty ones. We also want a wide diversity of different strains of bacteria to cover all the bases, so to speak. The gut contains many types of bacteria in different concentrations, depending on the person. There are 300-500 different types of microorganisms that can survive in the gut (Guarner 2003). Scientists are involved in many research projects currently to study the various strains of bacteria and how they affect us. For example, scientists have identified certain strains of bacteria as "fat" bacteria and other strains as "skinny" or "thin" bacteria – depending on how they react in your gut to promote or hinder your metabolism.

Your beneficial gut bacteria help with all sorts of vital functions in your body. They help with synthesizing vitamins. They help with protecting us from catching every disease that goes around. They help in controlling our appetite and sending a message when we are "full." They help with our natural healing system that we talked about in Chapter 1. The gut bacteria also help with regulating our hormones and our moods and even our blood pressure.

How do they do all this? The microbes (which include multiple categories of living organisms including bacteria) contain genes. The genes control many of the processes that occur throughout our digestive system. We want to turn on the genes that cause health and turn off the genes that cause disease. A Native American tale gives us some insight into how to do this.

The Tale of Two Wolves

A wise Cherokee Native American grandfather was talking to his grandchildren about life. As his grandchildren sat at his feet, he taught them using this story: He said, "I have a battle going on inside me. It is a ferocious fight between two strong wolves. One wolf is evil – he is angry and vicious and hateful. The other wolf is good – he is positive and helpful and loving. The two wolves are tangled in a great battle." The grandchildren thought about it for a while and then one asked, "Which wolf will win, Grandfather?" The wise grandfather replied, "Whichever wolf I feed."

That is exactly what we are going to start doing with our own microbiome. We are going to start feeding it the good stuff – whole fruits and veggies, fiber, healthy fats and beneficial bacteria.

Fecal Transplants

In just the last few years, a lifesaving treatment has come on the scene at a number of forward-thinking medical institutions in the U.S. Although this treatment has been performed in Europe for many years, it has only recently been gaining in popularity in the U.S. and is currently only approved for use in treating one illness. What treatment is this? Fecal transplants or FMT (Fecal Microbiota Transplantation). Fecal transplants are now approved for use in those suffering from *C. Diff.* – technically known as *Clostridium Difficile* Colitis- a very serious inflammation of the intestines caused by an overpopulation of the *C. Diff.* bacteria. This illness kills 14,000 Americans each year. In a fecal transplant, the feces in the digestive tract of someone healthy can be collected, filtered and placed by an enema-like process into a person with *C. Diff.* infection. The bacteria in the healthy feces begin to take hold in the colon of the person who is suffering with *C. Diff.* The healthy bacteria multiply and repopulate the colon. In a very short time of hours or days, the gut bacteria rebalances in the person, the person begins to feel better and their body gets back on track. This has a certain "*ewww*" factor, but when you consider that *C. Diff.* is a very serious infection which is often difficult to treat, usually requires hospitalization and can be deadly, suddenly, the fecal transplant sounds a lot more reasonable. (Not to mention, more reasonable in price than an expensive hospital stay with multiple courses of heavy-duty antibiotics.) Fecal transplants have a 90 percent cure rate when used for *C. Diff.* ("Quick, Inexpensive..." 2014). The New England Journal of Medicine published a study in 2013 demonstrating that fecal transplants were nearly twice as effective as antibiotics in treating *C. Diff.* Studies are currently underway to look at the possible use of fecal transplants in treating obesity, Irritable Bowel Syndrome, ulcerative colitis, celiac disease and even Parkinson's disease.

Mapping the Microbiome

Not surprisingly, when the stool samples of very sick people have been "mapped," they've been found to lack diversity in their microbial populations. A couple of strains of bacteria start to overpopulate the gut so that the variety that is needed for good health is compromised. The researchers started asking themselves – "what does a healthy microbiome look like?" They didn't know.

The National Institutes of Health (NIH) began The Human Microbiome Project – A $173 million, 5-year initiative. Launched in 2008, the study was to identify and characterize the microorganisms of a total of 300 healthy and unhealthy subjects. (Many other countries are now doing similar research. Lots of research dollars are going to study and "map" the human microbiome these days.)

But the NIH only studied 300 people at first. That's not enough to get a broad picture of what is going on in the general public.

Enter the American Gut Project.

The American Gut Project began when a guy named Jeff Leach (then a scientist at University of Colorado – Boulder) decided to "map" the gut bacteria of the general American population. He has now moved on to found the Human Food Project. Dr. Rob Knight and about 50 other collaborators are now continuing the important microbial research involved in mapping the gut bacteria of the general population. By using social media, they have piqued the interest of over 3,238 people ("Preliminary Characterization…" 2014) to get them to send in stool samples (along with other forms of a donation to the project). And in return, the donors receive a frame-able (no kidding) document in a color graph format that details which classes of microbes and in what proportions they have in the donated stool. Possibly because of its crowdsourcing and social media marketing strategy, the American Gut Project has samples from more people of varying ages than any other study of its kind. You can even "map" the microbiome of your pet.

Many agencies are currently involved in this type of microbiome research: the Biofrontiers Institute at the University of Colorado – Boulder and the Earth Microbiome Project at the University of Chicago as well as the Global Gut Project, to name a few.

The major Gut Bacteria Families are Firmicutes, which include Clostridium and Lactobacillus, among others, and Bacteroidetes, which includes Bacteroides and Prevotella, both of which break down polysaccharides (big sugars).

Can Our Microbiome Change?

Now, it turns out that stool samples differ dramatically depending on diet, age, and certain lifestyle factors, such as antibiotic usage and exercise. It has also been demonstrated that people from other parts of the world have a very different variety of microbes.

Many questions still need to be answered about why and how the gut microbiome changes. For now, at least, we are finding out that they *do* change and they can change quite quickly. And we know that it is possible to make changes to our diet to help facilitate these changes – both in positive and negative ways.

Taking a probiotic supplement adds billions of live organisms to our system, helping to support the populations of beneficial bacteria. Making sure we get lots of fiber from whole fruits and veggies every day helps boost the population of the "skinny" bacteria. You may have read about prebiotics – these are various types of non-digestible dietary fibers that activate the growth of beneficial bacteria. Eating small amounts of live cultures from yogurt, kefir, or fermented foods each day give support to the "good guys." Processed food and refined sugar feed the "fat" bacteria, so by limiting our intake of junk food and sweets, we keep the "fat" bacteria in check. Gluten is also a suspect in feeding some of the less beneficial bacteria. When our gut bacteria diversity is weak and out of balance, we can more easily acquire parasites, food-borne illness, and bacterial infections.

Gut Bacteria and Research

Recent research at the California Institute of Technology is looking at how gut bacteria play a role in autism. They are using autistic mice, which have, like many autistic people, a lack of diversity in their gut bacteria. By giving the autistic mice probiotics, they were able to change the balance of gut bacteria and the mice performed better on certain behavioral tests (Stoller-Conrad 2013).

Scientists have many theories on how the gut and brain interact. It is not well understood how our brain communicates with the gut bacteria, but it is clear that the bacteria play a role in our moods and brain activity and possibly even our cravings (Alcock 2014).

Recent research is shedding light on how hormones and gut bacteria are deeply intertwined. For example, two main hormones are involved in regulating our appetite. Grehlin, "the hunger hormone" and leptin, "the satiety hormone" work together to regulate your appetite. Without this system in good working order, your body keeps telling you you're hungry, even when you have just eaten. These hormones can be dramatically disrupted when the gut bacteria ecosystem is out of balance. Grehlin, the "hunger hormone" does not shut off after eating when the *H. pylori* gut bacteria is out of balance (Blaser 2011). Big problem! What happens when your body keeps telling you you're hungry? You keep eating. And eating. And eating. And guess what? That is exactly what a lot of us are doing. Maybe that is one of the reasons our obesity rate has been going up so dramatically in recent decades.

Gut bacteria are living organisms. They have to eat, too. Guess what they eat? They eat the fermented and partially digested food that is in your gut, for one. Now, that is pretty handy to have a healthy, happy ecosystem all feeding off of the calories you consume each day – if you have a diverse and healthy assortment of bacteria that are all living in harmony. Research has suggested that in the gut of someone with a healthy microbiome, the living organisms themselves, the gut bacteria, may consume about 450 kcal/day (a quarter of your calories) ("Fact: You Carry..." 2011). What happens in the gut of someone with a lack of diversity, or imbalance, in his or her gut bacteria? Their bacteria consume very small numbers of calories.

Research is being done looking at the connection between gut bacteria and heart disease. A study in 2013 has shown that gut bacteria in people who eat red meat produce a compound that may be contributing to heart disease (Koeth 2013).

Recent research shows that it could be your gut bacteria signaling your brain to crave a particular food (Alcock 2014). Could that be one of the nasty types trying to gain a foothold? Have you ever noticed that some people seem to be able to eat whatever they want in the quantity they want and not gain weight? Maybe this is due to their beneficial balance of gut bacteria.

September 5, 2013 New York Times:
Gut Bacteria From Thin Humans Can Slim Mice Down

A recent study showed that transplanting the gut bacteria from thin and obese human twins into thin mice had a dramatic result. The mice that received "thin bacteria" stayed thin. The mice that received "fat bacteria" got fat.

The Complex Problem

How are we supposed to fix all this? It's a complex problem. When you look at your situation, you may find many of these factors are contributing to your health issues. You may be craving addictive food and consuming too much junk food. In addition, your body's natural system that tells you to stop eating has been messed up so you overeat. Your gut bacteria may be out of balance and sluggish – creating a gut environment that is unhealthy. Then there's that hand sanitizer you've been using for years – it contains Triclosan that kills off the good bacteria along with the bad. Your stressful lifestyle upsets your digestive system. When you eat processed and sugary foods, they, in turn, feed those "fat" bacteria, resulting in weight gain. If you were born by C-section, you did not get the benefit of your mother's healthy bacteria going through the birth canal. Many of us were set on an unhealthy path to an unhealthy start in life for our microbiome. It can be overwhelming to try to resolve these complex issues.

The Solution

Well, a solution exists. It is not rocket science. Humans have been doing better at this gut bacteria thing for thousands of years. Our bodies want to be in balance. However, we've gotten ourselves off track. We need to give our gut some healthy boosts, limit the things that get it out of balance and get out of the way to let our natural body-balancing functions take over.

Researchers are honing in on how the differences in the gut bacteria affect our metabolism, our weight, and obesity. Scientists are studying the functions and byproducts of various strains of bacteria. Scientists are conducting studies to look at how the gut and brain communicate. We are beginning to understand how the diversity of bacteria can change and adapt over time and what that means for our health. Think about the story of the two wolves. It is time to quit feeding the evil wolf and start feeding the good wolf.

Chapter 7 has a detailed plan on how to begin to heal our digestive system, rebalance our microbiome and begin to get our gut back on track. The body responds quickly. Remember Jeff Leach, the guy who started the "American Gut Project?" He is spending a year trying different diets and living in different locations around the world to see just how fast the microbiome (as measured in fecal samples) can change. And the preliminary research shows – it can change in a matter of days!

What are you waiting for?

4| Warning: Gut Toxins Ahead

"The best way to detoxify is to stop putting toxic things into the body and depend upon its own mechanisms."

-Andrew Weil

Genetically Modified Organisms

Genetically Modified Organisms (GMOs) are foods that have been genetically altered by inserting a gene or multiple genes of one species into another species to give it very specific "programmed" qualities. This is dramatically different than cross breeding that has been practiced for thousands of years. Genetically altering a food makes it into a food that could never occur in nature – it often mixes animal with plant species. Now, this chapter is not about politics, laws or hype, so, put aside whatever opinions you have from the news and whatever ads you have seen on TV.

This chapter is about your body – remember, the one you own? This is about your gut. We have a growing body of research showing that animals fed a GMO diet suffer a wide range of health problems ranging from organ damage (Mesnag 2012) to massive tumors to fertility problems (including near complete sterility by the third generation of offspring in rats) (Smith 2003) to – you guessed it – intestinal damage (Samsel 2013). I fervently hope that GMOs in the diets of humans do not actually cause these problems and they are simply flawed studies. Since GMO's have not been tested long-term or on human subjects, and the U.S. allows production and sales of GM foods without labeling, we are essentially human guinea pigs. Many countries in the world ban or limit genetically modified foods, the U.S. being the biggest glaring exception. In the U.S. today, 70–80% of our foods contain genetically modified ingredients. If you think you are not eating GMOs, think again. Nearly every processed food contains GMOs. Nearly every restaurant uses foods that contain GMOs. It's not that there are a great multitude of GM crops, but rather, the crops that are GM are the most common ingredients used in processed foods in the U.S. – the oils, the sugars, the corn products and the soy products.

Serious Health Risks Associated With GMO Foods:

The American Academy of Environmental Medicine reported that, *"Several animal studies indicate serious health risks associated with GM food,"* including *infertility, immune problems, accelerated aging, faulty insulin regulation, and changes in major organs and the gastrointestinal system."*

In the U.S., the issues surrounding GMOs have become highly politicized. People have taken sides based on what they have heard in the media and ads they have seen on TV. Right now, for the purposes of this book, we are not concerned with the TV ads. For the moment, we don't care about labeling. We are concerned with your gut. If you are experiencing any of the symptoms discussed earlier having to do with digestive distress or health problems that can be due to digestive troubles, it could be because of gut damage caused by GMO foods that you are eating every day. There's a way to find out for yourself: try a Non-GMO diet. Many people who have started eating a non-GMO diet have started to feel almost instant relief from their digestive symptoms and other autoimmune symptoms. How do I eat a non-GMO diet, you might ask? It is difficult, in part, because the U.S. government does not require GMO foods to be labeled. But a growing number of concerned people are starting to take matters into their own hands. Here are some tips:

- Buy organic food. Certified Organic farmers are not allowed to knowingly plant GMO seeds. Products labeled 100% organic cannot intentionally include GMO ingredients. (Do not be fooled by the claim "all natural" which is not the same as organic and can contain GMO ingredients).

- Download the free iPhone app **ShopNoGMO** or consult the website *www.nonGMOShoppingGuide.com.*

- Look for products with either the "Non-GMO Project Verified" or the "Certified Organic" seal. Find out more at www.nongmoproject.org

- Do not eat processed food or restaurant food.

- Avoid the specific GMO foods and products that contain GMO ingredients.

Scientists have developed several types of technology used in GM crops and more are being developed. For example, corn is genetically engineered to be herbicide resistant and produce its own pesticide. Herbicide resistant GMO crops are made to survive repeated sprayings of a toxic broad-spectrum plant/weed killer that you may even have in your garage: RoundUp™. (The active ingredient in RoundUp™ is glyphosate.) Normally when you spray a plant in your yard with glyphosate, it dies. This is why you have it in your garage – to clear all plants from an area. Normally, if you spray it on your flowers or vegetables, they would die, too. The genetically modified crops do not die when sprayed. Instead, they are harvested and you eat them, along with the glyphosate residues that are on them. Recent research is linking glyphosate to the enormous increase of gluten sensitivity due to Leaky Gut Syndrome (Galland 2007).

Leaky Gut Syndrome is a gastrointestinal disorder in which the intestinal lining of the digestive tract becomes more permeable, or "leakier," than normal, due to repeated irritation and degrading of the gut lining, letting undigested proteins pass through.

The pesticide resistant GM crops work by producing Bt toxin – in essence, causing the plant to produce its own pesticide. Bt toxin kills specific classes of insects or larva by being incorporated into their digestive cell walls, creating pores.

When we eat the GMO foods, we are eating the toxic chemicals that are specifically designed to kill pests and weeds. And then they are inside us. The stomach breaks down almost all of these substances. The only problem is, some small amounts pass through the stomach, and then the "pests" and "weeds" that are under attack are our own gut bacteria and gut lining!

For people who are gluten sensitive (and experts now think that may be as many as 18 million Americans) symptoms of long-standing chronic conditions are often healed when gluten is removed from the diet. If you decide to go gluten-free, it would also be beneficial to try a GMO-free diet. The gluten and GMO foods in combination in the digestive system are both wreaking havoc. The GMO foods may be causing inflammation or leaky gut syndrome and damaging the lining, then the large gluten proteins escape through the more permeable gut and cause inflammation throughout the body. If you are getting rid of one in your diet, you might try giving up both for three weeks to see if you notice a reduction in your symptoms. If your symptoms do improve, then you now have a piece of the puzzle to help dramatically improve your health.

Which foods are GMO?

Corn and all corn products: Including cornstarch, high fructose corn syrup, corn oil and many corn-based ingredients.

Soybeans and all soy products: Including soymilk, soybean oil, tofu, many "meatless" products.

Vegetable oil: Since vegetable oil is not required to be produced from any particular source, it is a blend of oils and commonly contains the cheapest oils available – usually corn oil, soybean oil and cottonseed oil.

Canola oil: Canola oil is GMO and is often included in the vegetable oil blends.

Sugar (Sugar beets): Most sugar is made from sugar beets. It is the cheapest form of sugar. If a product says "pure cane sugar" is it NOT genetically modified but if it says simply "sugar" then chances are high it is GMO.

Meat and Dairy products: From animals that are fed GMO corn, alfalfa or soy-based feed.

Papaya (Hawaiian), Zucchini, Yellow summer squash: Also GMO crops.

Cottonseed: We don't eat cotton but it is a GM crop. And from it we get cottonseed oil that is often blended with other oils as an inexpensive source of fat in processed foods.

Alfalfa: We don't eat that either, but cows do and we, in turn, eat the beef.

Infant formula: Most are made from corn or soy.

Antibiotics

Antibiotics first became available in the late 1930's. In the whole history of human beings, that is not very long ago. The word antibiotics literally means "against life": "anti-bio." Granted, antibiotics have saved many lives. They are also routinely used to prevent and treat infection pre and post surgery, allowing many life-saving procedures to be carried out. We have come to think of many surgeries as "routine," "outpatient," and "not too serious." We have antibiotics to thank for much of that.

As we have heard in the mainstream media, antibiotic use has become so commonplace that it is losing its effectiveness. According to ("Antibiotic Prescribing…" 2011) U.S. children receive, on average, about 18 rounds of antibiotics before they are 18. For adults, the rate drops slightly to 4 rounds every 5 years ("Antibiotic Use Overview" 2010). Although the rate of antibiotic prescribing in children is going down (largely due to awareness about antibiotic overuse and resistance) it is still a common practice. Livestock are routinely given continuous doses of antibiotics en-mass just so they can survive the living and feeding conditions that they are subjected to. Did you know that 80% of the antibiotics sold in this country are fed or administered to livestock, which then become our food ("Most U.S. Antibiotics…" 2011)? All those antibiotics kill off helpful bacteria along with the less helpful bacteria.

Due to the overuse of antibiotics among other things, we now have antibiotic resistant bugs (mostly bacteria). Enter any hospital and you will find many practices that are followed simply to contain the spread of these superbugs that are very difficult to kill.

> **A World Health Organization report dated April 30, 2014**
> "This serious threat [of superbugs] is no longer a prediction for the future, it is happening right now in every region of the world and has the potential to affect anyone of any age, in any country. Antibiotic resistance – when bacteria change so antibiotics no longer work in people who need them to treat infections – is now a major threat to public health."

What did your grandparents do when they got sick?

They probably had a dozen reliable home remedies like peppermint oil, tea tree oil, lavender oil, homemade chicken soup (see recipe in Chapter 9), herbal tea, nasal rinses and poultices.

These days we seem to have forgotten many of these home remedies, and it's a shame. Many home remedies are very effective at relieving symptoms of common illnesses and promoting health and healing.

Today it seems many doctors treat each new health concern with yet another prescription medication. These medications and over the counter drugs all take a toll on our digestive system and our liver. But what you may not even think about is that the antibiotic that we may take so routinely for a cough or respiratory ailment actually may be doing permanent damage to our gut bacteria. It takes 6 months to a year[1] for your gut bacteria to get back in balance after a course of antibiotics. And some studies show that we might *never*, (yes, I said *never*) fully regain every type of friendly bacteria that were in our guts before taking the antibiotics (Blaser 2011).

---

[1] Different types of antibiotics have different effects.

The beneficial bacteria in your gut will normally keep the harmful bacteria under control. This process is not entirely understood, but it likely has to do with them competing for the same calorie sources. When the beneficial bacteria outnumber the harmful bacteria (as they should in a healthy, balanced gut) they gobble up more of the calories. When you take a course of antibiotics, the antibiotics destroy most of the strains of bacteria. Some of the harmful bacteria strains are antibiotic resistant. So they remain in the gut and begin to take over the sources of calories. Then the harmful bacteria become more plentiful.

Another thing that can happen is antibiotics can cause diarrhea. This is due to large numbers of beneficial bacteria dying off. With a bout of diarrhea, the intestinal tract is unable to maintain the proper ratio of beneficial bacteria to harmful bacteria. Nutrients do not get processed properly as they are flushed out of the body too quickly to be absorbed. The delicate balance of gut flora is flushed, literally, down the drain. The body has to replenish itself and this can take time. Meanwhile, your immune system is not functioning at its best level.

Yeast Infections and Leaky Gut Syndrome

One other way things get out of balance is through yeast over-growth, sometimes known as *Candida*. Many antibiotics do not kill the yeast (a fungus), only the bacteria. So, when a person takes a round of antibiotics that kills off most or all of the gut bacteria, the yeast that exists in the digestive tract has a chance to take over. It starts to grow like crazy, multiplying its forces. This is why some people will get yeast infections following a course of antibiotics. The yeast gets out of control without the beneficial bacteria to keep it in its place. Guess what the yeast "eats?" Sugar and foods that turn to "sugar" in the gut. And for many of us, there is plenty of that to go around to keep the yeast well fed!

Once the yeast gains a foothold, it starts to attack the gut walls and it causes inflammation. It creates sores or lesions in the delicate gut lining. This process, which can have multiple causes, is called leaky gut syndrome (see page 34). The digestive tract is its own tube to the outside world – it is designed to handle these larger food particles and outside substances. However, once you have holes in your gut, relatively large, partially digested food particles start to "leak" out into the bloodstream. Our internal environment doesn't recognize these "foreign particles". Our internal tissues and organs are not supposed to have to deal with large food particles – they only know how to deal with the microscopic nutrients once they have been absorbed into the bloodstream in the proper fashion. When you have undigested food and other substances floating around (in your blood, in your tissues, in your joints) where they shouldn't be, that triggers inflammation throughout the system. This can lead to all kinds of problems, including autoimmune diseases and all of the health problems associated with systemic inflammation.

It's time for a reboot.

If you or a family member does need to take antibiotics for a serious illness, you can begin the 21-Day Plan as soon as you begin to take the antibiotic. Studies have shown that taking the probiotics *during* the course of antibiotics leads to dramatically better outcomes and fewer side effects (Newberry 2012). A probiotic supplement will also help bring the gut back into balance more quickly after the antibiotics are finished. If you have taken antibiotics recently, or perhaps you suffer from leaky gut syndrome, yeast overgrowth or one of the other gut flora imbalances, you can take steps to heal and restore balance to your system.

5| Get Out of the Drive Thru Lane

"The thing about motorcycles is that it's nearly impossible to go through a drive thru. And eating fries is completely out of the question."

-Ryan Ross

I remember my first McDonald's hot fudge sundae. It was a new product at McDonald's, and my last day of 8th grade. I remember that particular McDonald's. It was near the mall. This was back when they had a sign below the golden arches that said 1 million served. I had eaten the cones before. But now the ice cream was in a little bowl with warmed fudge sauce on top.

Why do I remember that hot fudge sundae all these years later?

Perhaps because we didn't go to McDonald's very often. It was a rare treat. When we traveled, my mom packed sandwiches for the car. Our music lessons and sports were after school so we were all home by dinnertime. Hot lunch at school was cooked, not just reheated, by Mrs. Rucker.

Eating at fast food restaurants is no longer a rare treat. In fact, *"consumption of food prepared away from home plays an increasingly large role in the American diet. In 1970, 25.9 percent of all food spending was on food away from home; by 2012, that share rose to its highest level of 43.1 percent."* ("USDA ERS Home" 2014)

Fast Food Lifestyle

We eat a much higher percentage of our meals outside of the home now than we ever have. In fact, a hundred years ago, Americans ate 2% of their meals outside the home. Today, that number is 50%.

Meals eaten at fast food restaurants lead the statistics. According to the Pew Research Center, on 1/1/2014, there were 160,000 fast food restaurants in America, serving 50 million Americans every day.

USDA Economic Research Service:

A number of factors contributed to the trend of increased dining out since the 1970's, including a larger share of women employed outside the home, more two-earner households, higher incomes, more affordable and convenient fast food outlets, increased advertising and promotion by large foodservice chains, and the smaller size of U.S. households.

Processed Food

Our lifestyles have changed. The food itself has changed, too. Much of our food is very highly processed and contains many toxins. Toxins are damaging to your gut lining. The FDA maintains a list of the more than 3,000 additives, preservatives, flavorings and colorings that are added to foods in the U.S. ("Everything Added…" 2011). Ninety percent of our food budgets go to purchase the foods that have these types of ingredients.

Processed foods and fast foods contain a multitude of unrecognizable ingredients. For example, McDonald's McWrap™ contains 121 ingredients ("McDonald's McWraps…" 2013). McDonald's, Wendy's, Burger King, Carl's, Jr., and Pizza Hut all use an ingredient called azodicarbonamide. This ingredient is used as a dough conditioner and it is also used in producing yoga mats. Azodicarbonamide is banned in Europe and Australia. After intense U.S. media scrutiny in 2014, Subway restaurants in the U.S. removed this toxic chemical from their bread and Starbucks has announced that it will soon be removing it from their baked goods. Much of our food supply is manufactured on such a large scale that we have lost our connection to the source. One McDonald's burger, for example, contains the meat from more than 100 cows and is shipped frozen from thousands of miles away, to each restaurant ("Do McDonalds…" 2012).

Shocking statistics from Super Size Me website:

• French fries are the most eaten vegetable in the U.S.

• The average child sees 10,000 TV advertisements per year

• McDonald's distributes more toys per year than Toys-R-Us

• Before most children can speak, they can recognize McDonald's

---

It is amazing that we can feed our miraculous bodies such quantities of junk food, toxins and poisons and still, somehow our gut gets enough stuff to keep us going. Unfortunately, it can't keep us going forever. Eventually these toxins catch up with us. Just like Uncle Ray's belly. It may seem like everything is OK, but over time, the toxins build up in our tissues. Remember back when we talked about what your gut does with something it doesn't recognize? It sticks it in fat tissues to get it out of the way, so it can deal with the more important process of absorbing the needed nutrients. Once we reach a certain level of toxicity, we may develop conditions such as low energy, aches and pains, weight gain, or we easily catch colds, infections, and respiratory ailments. Or worse - we may develop autoimmune diseases, heart disease or Type 2 diabetes.

When this happens, our body is not running at its optimal level.

What's needed? We need a little more attention to the care and feeding of our digestive systems.

Food Addictions

The fact is many of us are actually addicts – food addicts, sugar addicts. That sounds strong but it is human nature to seek pleasure and avoid pain. Many foods that are available to us are biologically addictive. Sugar is 8 times as addictive as cocaine, according to a 2007 study (Magalie 2007). Dr. Mark Hyman has a name for soda: liquid death. We have all succumbed to the craving to grab our favorite junk food and stuff ourselves silly.

The fast food restaurants are in business to make money. The food industry is a trillion dollar a year industry. Anytime we are talking about that enormous amount of money, there are going to be some big, powerful players who are going to be doing everything in their power to hang onto market share. They are not in business to help you stay healthy. The foods they offer are highly processed and contain addictive substances. Part of the problem is corporations have mastered the art of marketing. They have hijacked our health and our children's health. Did you know that the U.S. is one of only a handful of countries that allows food marketing directly to kids?

Are there healthy options in the drive thru? Maybe a few – the salads, the yogurt, the oatmeal. But once you pull up, you want the fries and soda, too. And even if you can resist, your kids can't. They want their free toy!

Your cravings for fast food and processed food will subside when you have your gut in balance and you are filling your body with good nutrition. I am not saying it is easy to stop going to the drive thru, but if you do, your gut will certainly thank you.

Small Changes, Big Differences

If we start to really think about putting in more good stuff and less bad stuff, it will make a big difference. We don't have to change everything overnight. If we make sure we are getting plenty of water plus fiber in the form of whole fresh fruits and green vegetables, our gut runs more smoothly and it is able to process things better. And if we take a little time each day to walk or exercise or move our body in some way, all of our systems, gut included, will function better. And all these things, plus the magnesium citrate at bedtime, will help us get a good night's sleep as well. How do you feel when you get a good night's sleep? Hormonally, your body – and your gut – is in better balance so that you feel fewer cravings, you are more even tempered, you are more energetic, and more motivated to do whatever it is you love to do!

6| Your Sensitive System: Every Body is Different

"Your body will be around a lot longer than that expensive handbag. Invest in yourself." — Pinterest

What is Wellness?

I was at a happy hour networking event and a guy asked me about this book. He asked what diet is best of all the diets. I explained that I thought different diets work well for different people – no one diet will work well for everyone. I said, "For example, some people do well on a Paleo diet and others do well on a vegan diet."

The Paleo diet: Often called the caveman diet, based on foods that were available in the Paleolithic era – before modern agriculture, processed foods and dairy were available. Diet is comprised of meat from free-range or wild caught animals, lots of vegetables and fruits, plenty of high quality fats and very little processed or refined foods.

The Vegan diet: A diet that excludes all animal products including meat, eggs, dairy and any ingredients that contain animal products.

Then he said, "What do you mean by, "do well?" That got me thinking. How do we know if we are doing well? What is the definition of "doing well?"

> **Wellness:** The state or condition of being in good physical and mental health.

If you "Feel Good," as James Brown used to say, is that doing well? Well, if you wake up in the morning with plenty of energy to get through your day – seems to me, that is "doing well." If you do not need to rely on drugs: caffeine, sugar, alcohol, cigarettes, other drugs – to "keep going," that seems like it should at least be *part* of the definition of doing well. If you are doing more than just surviving – if you feel that, physically, you are thriving, then would you say you are doing well? I would. Mental health is part of the equation, too. In order to have the sense that you are doing well, you would want to have a feeling of satisfaction with the emotional and social aspects of your life.

Obstacles to Wellness:

Constipation

Imagine if your garbage disposal clogged up and your kitchen sink wasn't draining. You didn't have time to deal with it, so you kept dumping things down the drain. You turned the switch of the disposal on and off, on and off. It gurgled, but all that gunk still remained – the sink was still clogged. Well, you were out the door to work, so, it would have to wait until later. You came home – still clogged. Add the dinner leftovers and scrape the dog's dish into the drain. Still clogged. Now it has turned into a gross, stinky mess. Get the picture?

Well, you can't expect to read a book on digestion and gut health without talking at least a little bit about "poop," which is a word less disagreeable than feces. So, to keep everything in tiptop working order, we need to be pooping at least once a day. Minimum. If you poop more often, fine. If you poop less often than once a day, listen up. If you do not poop at least once a day, your garbage disposal (digestive tract, that is) backs up, gets clogged and cannot do its job. Not only that, everything inside gets even more stuck, making it harder and harder to "go." All those toxins that your body was ready to get rid of are instead at a standstill, stuck inside you – just like a traffic jam on the freeway. This is a recipe for disaster.

John, age 81, reported that after completing the 21-Day Plan his constipation went from a 7 (moderately severe symptoms) to a 3 (mild symptoms). Prior to starting the 21-Day Plan, he reported that he had moderately severe gas (9 on a scale of 1 to 10) and his gas was dramatically decreased (4 on a scale of 1 to 10) at the end of 21 days. His insomnia also improved from an 8 (moderately severe insomnia) to a 6 (moderate insomnia) in just 21 days. In addition, his fatigue level fell from a 10 (severe fatigue) to a 6 (moderate fatigue) on a scale of 1 to 10. He describes his experience this way: *"Easy to follow and I am feeling better."*

There are gentle, natural ways to clean out "the drain" so to speak. One thing that can help is a mild dose of magnesium citrate at bedtime. Magnesium is one of the minerals that allow the muscle cells to relax. This helps on so many levels, to calm and soothe the digestive system, loosen up those muscles that are tight from stress and relax all of the organs. It helps calm the nervous system to ensure a good night's sleep. And a good night's sleep allows the digestion to rest and heal to get ready for the next day. A low magnesium level can also be linked to depression, so making sure you are getting enough of this important mineral is very helpful for that "feeling good" daily energy.

Food Sensitivities and Food Allergies

Many people have food sensitivities and allergies and are not aware of them. Food sensitivities and food allergies are different. An actual food allergy is an immune system response to eating the food. That particular food will always trigger the same immune system response. The most common foods that people are allergic or sensitive to are dairy (especially cow's milk), wheat/gluten, soy, eggs, citrus, corn, nightshades, peanuts, fish, shellfish, and tree nuts.

> Susie, 51, often has a reaction after eating certain foods – clearing her throat and mild sniffles. She completed the 21-Day Plan and reported that her allergic response went from a 5 (moderate allergic response) to a 3 (mild allergic response) following the 21-Day Plan

A food sensitivity or intolerance is more general and can vary. This can be because the body lacks the enzymes needed to digest the food properly or there may be other reasons that a person is not able to process a food. People may develop an uncomfortable reaction to the food; however, it is not an immune response. It could be a variety of symptoms such as yawning and feeling tired immediately after eating a food or digestive disturbances such as gas or bloating, headaches or migraines. Symptoms may be subtle and sometimes symptoms are delayed 24 to 48 hours after eating the food.

Once you determine your allergies and/or sensitivities, by focusing more specifically on discovering and avoiding their source, you will begin to feel much better when you stop eating the offenders. It requires paying close attention to what your Inner Doctor is saying.

Inflammation

Our body needs an environment that is not inflamed to be at its best. A steady diet of fried, processed foods, and sugar has made many of us in a constant state of chronic inflammation. Think about inflammation for a minute. What if you jam your finger? It swells up almost instantly. It is painful to move it. This is your body's way of healing – making you rest it to give it time to heal. That's one purpose of inflammation. But many of us have chronic inflammation all over our bodies, all the time. Think of that jammed finger on a larger scale. What if your body is giving you mandatory rest all day, every day due to chronic, systemic inflammation? No wonder we don't feel like we have any energy! We want our digestive tract (and our whole body) to be calm, cool and collected, not hot, angry and swollen, in order to take care of business. Many of the things we will learn about in Chapter 7 will help develop the non-inflammatory environment – the lemon juice in the morning with water, the mug of home-brewed green tea, the magnesium citrate and the whole fruits and vegetables.

Putting Your Best Foot Forward
Tips for Digestive Wellness

If the digestive system is not "doing well" then it is unlikely that you are feeling your best. What does your gut need – or want – to be at its best? Again, think about what makes you feel good at your gut level. Picture your gut as a long, narrow tube with lots of twists and turns. Your job is to make many things move through the tube everyday – from the top to the bottom. What would help in the process?

Water

The first thing is water. We need lots of water to keep everything flowing – literally! Start each day with a glass of water right when you wake up in the morning. If you like, add the juice of half a lemon (see more in Chapter 7). Your system has been repairing and replenishing during the night. Time to put some water back into the tract. This has the added benefit of activating your kidneys, as well.

Fiber From Fruits and Veggies

Next up, fiber. We depend on a certain amount of roughage to thicken things up so everything has enough bulk to keep on moving. The best sources of fiber come from fresh, whole fruits and veggies. A morning smoothie made with frozen blueberries and banana goes a long way to adding some roughage into the tract. Your large serving of green veggies that is recommended in the 21-Day Plan also provides roughage and plenty of micronutrients!

Chewing Your Food Well

One tip for good digestion is to chew your food thoroughly before swallowing. Sounds simple, but many of us don't do it. The enzyme ptyalin is released in your mouth as you chew which begins breaking down the food so it is partially digested even by the time it hits your stomach. Eating fast without taking the time to chew your food thoroughly also can trigger acid reflux.

Micronutrients

If you are trying to improve your digestion and give your body the nourishment it needs, you want to get plenty of micronutrients. I am sure you have heard of the macronutrients – Fats, Carbs and Protein. The micronutrients are the vitamins, minerals, and phytochemicals that are found in high concentrations in fruits, vegetables, seeds and nuts. Many of these nutrients have been analyzed and named, such as beta-carotene. Others are still being discovered. These micronutrients are what your cells are hungry for to make all of your systems function with full energy and vitality. Dr. Joel Fuhrman writes about micronutrients and the nutrient-density of foods in his book *Eat For Health*. He notes, *"In the last 50 years, there have been over 10,000 experiments showing the value of consuming high-nutrient plant foods."* Guess how many micronutrients are found in a bagel with cream cheese? Almost none. A steak? Very few. A burger and fries? Practically zero. (A few if you add tomato and lettuce.) A frozen waffle with butter and syrup? Zippo. A big, green salad with several, colorful veggies? TONS!

Micronutrients: Nutrients required by humans and other organisms throughout life in small quantities to orchestrate a range of physiological functions.

You now have everything flowing through regularly, emptying waste daily; things are functioning well. Now the body is ready to take in all those wonderful micronutrients. Actually, you have been absorbing some micronutrients all along. But now that you are pooping every day, you will have a nice fresh slate that will be ready for some good, healthy absorption. Your cells need vitamins and minerals. Your muscles need vitamins and minerals. Your brain needs vitamins and minerals. Get the picture? Get yourself plenty of good fruits, veggies, seeds, nuts and whole foods. All of the functions of your daily activities require energy and good functioning muscles and a quick brain. Micronutrients will give you the special boost you need for sports performance, energy and enthusiasm for life.

Enzymes

What are enzymes? These compounds found in fresh fruit and veggies aid in the digestion process, breaking down the foods for better absorption. On the 21-Day Plan we get enzymes from fresh squeezed lemon juice and fresh fruit and veggies. Our body can also make some enzymes itself if it has all the necessary raw materials. Many people also find it helpful to take a digestive enzyme supplement to boost their digestive processes.

> **Enzymes:** a substance produced by a living organism that acts as a catalyst to bring about a specific biochemical reaction.

Fermented Foods

Fermented foods. Ever heard of those? Many fermented foods have probiotics *and* fiber – a powerhouse of goodness for your gut. These foods are somewhat strange to us, but they are great for gut healing. People have been eating fermented foods in many cultures for over 5,000 years. Fermented foods, simply put, are foods that are produced or preserved by the action of microorganisms. The sugars interact with the food and turn into something else. The food is partially broken down in this process, making it easier to digest. The fermented foods also contain the "good stuff" that your gut bacteria like to eat-bacteria that we want to promote in our system. By eating fermented foods we replenish and maintain the diversity of our gut bacteria. Fermented foods include kefir (yogurt-type drink), sauerkraut, miso, tempeh, fermented vegetables such as kimchi, pickles and many other sour or pickled foods. The best ones for gut health will be sold in the refrigerated section (not the shelves) of the grocery store to keep the cultures alive. You might want to try making your own at home. Other fermented foods include sourdough bread, kombucha (a fermented beverage), wine and beer. A little goes a long way in fermented food land. Just a small serving of fermented vegetables, for example, added to a salad or entrée regularly is enough to benefit your gut.

Definitions:

Kefir: A milk drink with old origins thought to be in Northwestern Asia, made by fermenting milk (all types) with a combination of yeast and bacteria (which form microbial colonies called "grains").

Miso: A Japanese seasoning made by fermenting soybeans with salt and a particular fungus (*kōjikin*). Often used as we might use a soup bouillon – spooning a small amount of miso paste into hot water for soup.

Tempeh: A fermented whole soybean product originating from Indonesia that is pressed into various shaped patties and aged. Can be used in stir-fries or marinated and grilled. Often used as a meat substitute.

Kimchi: A traditional aged, fermented Korean side dish made with a variety of vegetables (often including cabbage) that is both spicy and sour.

Now you may be asking, "Is wine fermented?" Yes. So is beer. "Whoo-hoo. I am all set," you may be thinking. There have been many studies demonstrating that one or two servings of alcohol per day can have health benefits. The key is to listen to your body.

People have different levels of tolerance for alcohol. Alcohol can interfere with sleep. It can interfere with other good health intentions, such as portion control of foods eaten at the same time. And alcohol can be toxic. They don't call it "intoxicated" for nothing. Obviously, too much alcohol can have disastrous health effects. By paying close attention to your body and the signals, you may be able to enjoy the healthy benefits of reasonable amounts of fermented wine and beer.

Elimination Diet

You may need to experiment to find which foods are causing allergies or sensitivities. One way to figure out your "offenders" is to do an elimination diet. This is something you can do at home – no blood work required. A quick online search will give you many elimination diet plans to choose from. Choose one that eliminates the most common food sensitivities, such as the Elimination Diet Printable One-Sheet from www.doctoroz.com.

During an elimination diet, you restrict your diet to foods that are known to *not* trigger allergic responses in most people. During the time you choose for your elimination diet, you avoid eating the foods that are known to cause reactions in many people. Three weeks is the suggested time frame to let your body clear out all of the traces of the foods that trigger your issues. Many people will have a dramatic decrease in their symptoms. Then comes the somewhat challenging task of "testing" each of the potential allergens, one by one, to discover which are the culprits. Once you determine which food(s) you are sensitive to, you can add back in the other foods and resume a normal diet – minus the offender. Going through this process with the assistance of a health coach or healthcare practitioner who is experienced in elimination diets can be very beneficial as you may want support and a guiding voice when you have questions.

My husband, Doug, suffered severe asthma since the age of 4. Growing up, he felt unable to participate in physical activities or sports because any exercise would trigger an asthma attack. He made many trips to the Emergency Room over the years for lifesaving medications to bring the attacks under control. As an adult he took advantage of newer medications to manage his disease, but he did not have his asthma under control. In 1999, at the urging of his holistic doctor, he tried a three-week elimination diet. Skeptical is not a strong enough word to describe how he felt about the idea that food allergies might cause the asthma he had suffered with his whole life. Boy, was he shocked when before the three weeks were even over, his asthma attacks and his wheezing were dramatically reduced! It took several more weeks to determine exactly which foods triggered the asthma and several more months until he was able to reduce and ultimately eliminate his use of all asthma medication (with his doctor's supervision). Today, he does not take any asthma medication and has no asthma symptoms. He continues to avoid his trigger foods and completely controls the asthma through diet.

Asking Good Questions

Take a few minutes to answer this question: "What is my body hungering for?" If you often have cravings for sugar, caffeine, alcohol, fried food, salty food, soda, or any other food that does not have much in the way of nutritional value, it can be valuable to figure out the causes of your cravings. Cravings can be triggered by many things such as a lack of certain nutrients, dehydration, an imbalance of hormones or cravings can be a response to emotions such as stress or boredom. Cravings can also become a habit – an unhealthy part of your regular routine every day – such as a candy bar at your desk every day at 4:00 pm. Many cravings are simply due to the addictive nature of the foods and food additives themselves. Joshua Rosenthal writes extensively about cravings in his book, *Integrative Nutrition – Feed Your Hunger for Health and Happiness.* Bringing awareness to what foods you crave and why you might crave those particular foods is the first step to making healthier choices. The following questions will begin to help you work your way through the layers of your cravings and the foods you may be addicted to and get to a solution – identifying the real, nutritious food that your body needs to thrive!

What am I craving that I know is not nutritious?

What is my body hungering for that is nutritious?

What do I know my body needs to thrive?

When you ask yourself "What does my body need to thrive?" maybe your answer is not a food at all. Perhaps you need more sleep or less stress or more exercise. Don't worry. We will get to those topics in the next few chapters.

What is my body telling me to *stop* eating?

When our family gathered last Christmas, I was talking to my brother over cocktails and appetizers and we were talking about digestion and the topics in this book.

My brother said, "You're going to tell me to stop eating cheese, aren't you?"

I replied, "No. I would not tell you to stop eating cheese, unless *you think* your body would be better off without cheese."

He thought for a moment and said, "I guess I probably need to stop eating cheese."

When we take a few minutes to think it through, we often realize that we already know what would make us feel better.

I know what you are thinking: This book promised that you would not have to give up your favorite foods "cold turkey." You don't have to. You *can* make significant improvements to your digestion without eliminating any foods. The 21-Day Plan will give you positive benefits without giving up anything. But for many of you, after following the 21-Day Plan, you are going to have more energy and feel great. With better nutrition, you will begin to crave more of the good things and less of the bad. You are going to feel so good that you will want to increase *all* of your options to feel as good as you possibly can.

Healing Crisis

Occasionally, people begin to make healthy changes such as the recommendations in this book and they feel *worse* before they feel better. This is often referred to as a healing crisis. As the body flushes out the stored toxins and gets used to new foods and routines, the organs can sometimes get overwhelmed. For some people, this can cause 2-3 days of nausea, headaches, and fatigue. If symptoms can be managed during this period while continuing the healthy changes and the body is given time to rest, most people experience renewed energy and vitality once the healing crisis is over.

Benefits of good daily routine

For many of us, having a daily routine is helpful to keep our delicate systems on their game. The good habits become just that – habits. The things we do in any given day we are more likely to do again the next day. It's human nature. When we do make changes that help us feel better, we want to keep them up. I like to write or type up my daily routine. The actions you put energy into take on a more important role. I print out my ideal healthy daily routine and post it near my desk or by my bathroom mirror. I glance through it regularly to remind myself to focus my energy on those healthy actions.

Template for Daily Healthy Routine

What time do I wake up?

How do I get my day off to a good start?

Breakfast that gets my day going right:

When do I plan to get my exercise in today?

What is my exercise plan for today?

What healthy foods do I want to eat today?

If I get off-track today, what can I do to get back on board?

What will I do today to take care of myself?

What is my best bedtime to get a good night's sleep?

PART TWO
7| Take Action: The 21-Day Plan

"All roads lead to the gut."

- Mark Sisson

So here we are. Time for the 21-Day Plan, now that we know the critical role our gut plays in our health.

It's time to take action. This plan is designed to start slowly, adding small action steps over the course of the three weeks. The plan is easy to follow and contains enough detail and description for you to be able to acquire and eat the right things at the right times. The 21-Day Plan is designed to take only a small amount of time each day so that you only need to make minor adjustments to your daily schedule or lifestyle. What makes this plan different from many others is that it's designed to *add-in* foods and supplements to your diet, rather than make you *stop* eating particular foods. Joshua Rosenthal introduces the concept of *adding-in* good foods and *crowding-out* bad foods in his book, *Integrative Nutrition – Feed Your Hunger for Health and Happiness.*

What to Expect on the 21-Day Plan for Better Digestion and Increased Energy:

* More water everyday
* Meet your new breakfast smoothie
* More fiber and nutrients every day in the form of whole fruit and green veggies
* Start the day with a glass of water with lemon juice to "set the stage" for good   digestion all day – alkalinizes the body
* Add in fermented foods
* Green tea everyday – for antioxidants and anti-inflammatory properties
* Probiotic live cultures – through yogurt and probiotic supplement
* Magnesium citrate at bedtime to calm the body for good sleep and good digestion
* Move your body everyday

As you make changes, adding in foods and supplements, pay attention to the signals your body is sending.

What to look for:

* Changes in digestion
* Changes in stool
* Changes in sleep
* Changes in appetite
* Changes in energy
* Changes in symptoms such as pain, headaches, acid reflux, skin rashes, arthritis, etc.
* Changes in weight
* Changes in mood
* Changes in cravings

This plan contains advice and information relating to health care. It should be used to supplement rather than replace the advice of your doctor or other trained health professional. If you know or suspect that you have a health problem, it is recommended that you seek your physician's advice before embarking on any medical program or treatment. All efforts have been made to assure the accuracy of the information contained in this plan as of the date of printing. The author, editor and publishing company disclaim liability for any medical outcomes that may occur as a result of applying the methods suggested in this plan.

The 21-Day Plan for Better Digestion and Increased Energy

Beginning Date of my 21-Day Plan	
Ending Date of my 21-Day Plan	

Section One:

Complete this section *before beginning the plan.*

We now know, 70% of our immune system is in the gut. So, many of the health issues and symptoms you experience all over your body can be caused by poor gut conditions. Therefore, you want to measure your symptoms before and after you complete the plan to note any changes.

Mark on the scale of 1 to 10 how you experience the following symptoms:

	None	Moderate	Severe
Respiratory issues	1	5	10
Known environmental allergies	1	5	10
Skin Issues	1	5	10
Itchy eyes/watery eyes	1	5	10
Known food allergies	1	5	10

	None	Moderate	Severe
Muscle weakness	1	5	10
Arthritis pain/joint pain	1	5	10
Muscle pain	1	5	10
General aches and pains	1	5	10
Leg cramps/foot cramps	1	5	10
Headaches/migraines	1	5	10
Low energy level/fatigue	1	5	10
Irritable/mood swings	1	5	10
Insomnia/poor sleep quality	1	5	10
Not waking up rested	1	5	10
Constipation	1	5	10
Diarrhea/loose stools	1	5	10
Gas	1	5	10
Belching	1	5	10
"Rock in stomach" feeling	1	5	10
Indigestion/Heartburn/Reflux	1	5	10
Bad Breath	1	5	10

	Mild	Moderate	Severe
Overweight	1	5	10
Underweight	1	5	10

Other symptoms that may be related to digestion (please list):

What are your goals? What health issues are you hoping to address?

Describe your stress level currently:

Do you experience brain fog/memory issues?

List any blood sugar issues.

How is your immunity? Do you catch colds easily?

How would you describe your energy level, in general?

How would you describe your appetite?

Do you crave sugar, coffee, alcohol or cigarettes? Which do you consume on a regular basis?

How would you describe your health, in general?

In your own words, describe how you feel as you are beginning the 21-Day Plan?

The 21-Day PLAN: Overview

Week One: Setting the Stage for Good Digestion

Each day of Week One:

1) First thing in the morning, squeeze half a lemon into 12 oz. of water (room temp water is fine – whatever water you normally drink). Drink this before you eat or drink anything else in the morning.

2) Measure ¼ cup of organic yogurt or kefir (yogurt-type drink) and eat or drink this every day. It's not a large quantity – a small quantity every day over time, maintains the healthy gut bacteria levels. Add it to your smoothie for convenience, if you like.

3) Eat a breakfast smoothie every morning for healthful nutrients and fiber. Use the New Breakfast Smoothie Recipe, Chocolate

Cherry Smoothie from recipe chapter or use the smoothie template on page 80. Feeling creative? Make your own smoothie using at least one cup of fruit, non-dairy liquid, some protein to keep you going and little or no added sweetener.

New Breakfast Smoothie Recipe:

- 1 cup frozen blueberries
- 1/3 or 1/2 banana, frozen in chunks (see note below)
- 5 walnut halves
- ¼ cup organic yogurt (optional)
- ¼ tsp. cinnamon
- approx. 2/3 cup unsweetened almond milk

Add all ingredients except almond milk to blender. Add almond milk up to 16 oz. mark. Blend until smooth and creamy.

Week Two: Adding in good bacteria and antioxidants

Each day of Week Two:

Complete the action steps in Week One PLUS:

1) In addition to smoothie, eat one serving of whole, raw fruit every day. Alternate between bananas, apples, pears and 1 cup of fresh berries, such as strawberries or blueberries.

2) Probiotic capsule (see FAQ for recommended types) taken with a 12 oz. glass of water. Please do not take your probiotic capsule with a *hot* beverage as it can damage the live organisms in the supplement.

3) Drink a mug of green tea. (Note: Green tea has a mild level of caffeine. Drink green tea earlier in the day so sleep is not disrupted.)

Week Three: Adding in magnesium citrate, green vegetables, and exercise

Each day of Week Three:

Complete the action steps from Weeks One and Two *plus*:

1) Eat a large serving of green vegetables every day. This can be eaten whenever it is convenient for you – at lunch or dinner or even for a snack. The green vegetables can be cooked or raw or in a garden salad. Add ¼ cup of fermented veggies to your green veggies when you are eating at home.

2) Add in some movement/exercise to your day. If you are not active, find a time that is convenient for a short walk. If you are physically active, continue your regular exercise routine and add a short walk on days when you do not do your regular exercise.

3) At bedtime every night, take the recommended dose of magnesium citrate powder, stirred into a *small* (approx. 4 oz.) glass of water. Alternatively, you may take magnesium citrate in capsule form. Drinking a large glass of water at bedtime is not recommended if it causes you to wake in the night to use the bathroom.

Shopping List for 21-Day Plan

You can find a printer-friendly version at www.gutguide101.com, or see the resource section for a one-page tear-out version.

Purchase the two supplements (probiotic capsule and magnesium citrate) before beginning the plan. Purchase the first week's supply of groceries before beginning the plan. Restock fruits and veggies, as needed every few days.

Grocery Store – Week One:

_____4 lemons

_____Smoothie Supplies

_____Organic yogurt or kefir (enough for 7 small servings)

Health Food Store/Drugstore/Online – One shopping trip for the whole 21-Day Plan:

_____ Probiotic supplement, at least 14 capsules

_____ Natural Calm™ Magnesium Citrate supplement, 8 oz. jar

Grocery Store – Week Two:

_____Box of green tea bags or green tea/fruit blend tea bags, at least 14 bags

_____4 lemons

_____2 bananas

_____2 apples

_____2 pears

_____2 servings of fresh strawberries or blueberries

_____Organic yogurt or kefir (enough for 7 small servings)

Grocery Store – Week Three:

_____4 lemons

_____2 bananas

_____2 apples

_____2 pears

_____2 servings of fresh strawberries or blueberries

_____Organic yogurt or kefir (enough for 7 small servings)

_____Broccoli or green beans or leafy greens or ingredients for small garden salads, enough for 7 large servings

_____Sauerkraut or kimchi or other fermented vegetables (found in refrigerated aisle)

Frequently Asked Questions

Q: How does the 21-Day Plan work?

A: It is divided into Week 1, Week 2, and Week 3. Each week has three things that you do every day. The things you begin in Week 1 continue through Weeks 2 and 3, so in Week 3 you will be incorporating _all nine_ of the new habits from all three weeks. The Plan is designed to have foods and supplements _added in_ to your regular diet. You do not need to give up your favorite foods, your morning coffee or your favorite cocktail to follow this plan. You may eat at restaurants. Many people resist following a plan altogether if they are told they need to give up something they love. The theory behind _Gut Guide 101_ is that it is possible to improve digestion and increase energy levels without giving up the things you love.

Q: Which day should I start?

A: Look at your calendar and choose which 21-day period you will choose to do the program. Some people like to go get the supplies and start tomorrow. Great! Some like to look ahead and avoid certain weeks that are very busy or stressful. If you have any travel coming up, you may want to work around that. It is certainly possible to take the needed items with you when traveling; however, often when trying to follow a program, it is easier when you are at home and can work the plan into your regular routine. If you need to, it is OK to split up the 21 days, however, your results will likely be better if you are able to do 21 consecutive days.

Q: What do I need to buy?

A: Take the shopping list to the grocery store for the food items. You will also need to go to a health food store or drugstore to purchase the supplements, or they can both be purchased online at www.vitacost.com. You will need to check your supply of fruits and veggies every few days and make additional trips to the store as needed to make sure you have the whole fruits and green veggies for the next day.

Q: What if I have concerns about medications I am taking?

A: Please talk to your doctor if you have any medical concerns or if you have any reason to believe that any part of this program might not be right for you. Please talk to your doctor or pharmacist if you have any concerns with any medications you are taking or any of the supplements suggested in the program. If you notice any adverse effects, please stop the 21-Day Plan and contact your doctor, if necessary.

Q: I am taking a blood thinner. Do I need to be careful about the green veggies?

A: Some green veggies (especially dark leafy greens) and green tea have a high level of Vitamin K. When taking a blood thinner you may have been advised to limit your Vitamin K intake. Please talk to your doctor or your dietician about which green veggies would be best for you. Also ask if you need to check your blood work (INR) more frequently during the 21-Day Plan.

Q: What if I miss a day on the 21-Day Plan?

A: If you do get "off track" and you miss a day of the 21-Day Plan, that is OK. Sometimes you forget or you get busy or you get overwhelmed. It is quite common that you might miss one day. It is perfectly normal for this to happen when you are changing your routine. Simply try to jump back in and follow the program the next day. If you forget for several days, you may want to add some days at the end of the program so that you get the benefits of the whole 21-Day Plan.

Q: What if I already do some of these things every day?

A: That's great! Keep up the healthy habits you have already established. For example, if you already eat green veggies every day, then certainly continue that, throughout the three weeks and beyond. Think of the 21-Day Plan as a helpful guide to add healthy habits to your daily routine. Taking this time to focus daily on improving your digestion is new for many people. It takes time to reorganize your daily routine. Most people find it easier to make a few small changes at a time, rather than *all nine* changes at once. That is why the recommendations are phased in over three weeks. Furthermore, if you do notice that your digestion is improving and you have more energy, or maybe you are sleeping better or one of more of your symptoms have improved, you are encouraged to continue these changes beyond the 21 days. The actions that are recommended in the 21-Day Plan are great to incorporate into your daily life on a long-term basis, to maintain good digestion and better health.

Q: Can I make substitutions for the recommended foods, such as: frozen fruit, bottled lemon juice or Go-gurt™?

A: In general, attempt to eat the most whole, fresh version of the food that you can find. However, life happens. For various reasons, we have to make compromises in life. Decide what your goal is. For the 21-Day Plan, getting some nutrients into your body is ultimately the goal. If it is a matter of not eating the item at all or eating a less-than-ideal version, eat the less-than-ideal version. This is Gut Guide 101, after all. It's not a graduate level course.

Q: What are fermented foods? See page 54

A: Fermented foods, simply put, are foods that are produced or preserved by the action of microorganisms. These would include kefir (yogurt drink), sauerkraut, miso soup, tempeh, fermented vegetables such as kimchi, pickles and many other sour or pickled foods. You can find kimchi and fermented vegetables in the refrigerated pickle section of your grocery store. These foods contain gut-friendly bacteria. By eating them we replenish and maintain the diversity of our gut bacteria. Just a small serving of about ¼ cup of fermented vegetables or sauerkraut added to something else such as a salad or side dish is enough to benefit your gut. If you are watching your sodium levels, check your labels. Many pickled items are high in sodium.

Q: What if I don't like the foods?

A: There is a lot of flexibility in the suggested foods. The program includes one piece or serving of fresh whole fruit, every day during Week 2 and Week 3. Beginning in Week 3, you will be adding a large serving of green veggies every day. These are included for fiber and nutrients. For the fruit, I am recommending alternating between whole bananas, whole raw apples, pears and one cup of fresh berries, such as strawberries. If you dislike one of those fruits or you run out one day, then substitute another fruit you enjoy. I suggest alternating these to get a variety of gut-friendly benefits over the 21 days and to keep it interesting.

During Week 3, we add one large serving of green vegetables every day. I recommend either a large serving of steamed green vegetables such as broccoli or green beans or leafy greens or a side garden salad or spinach salad. Keep in mind the goal is to get a large serving of *green* vegetables – either cooked or raw is fine. If you choose a salad which is mostly cheese and croutons and ranch dressing on a small serving of iceberg lettuce, you will not be getting the full benefit of the fiber and nutrients that is beneficial for digestion. If you normally like your green veggies with a sauce or seasoning or dressing, that is fine. The goal is to eat green veggies every day, however you enjoy them is up to you.

Q: Why the lemon juice every day?

A: A 12 oz. glass of room temp water with juice of half a lemon squeezed in is a great way to start the day. The digestion works best when it is more alkaline than acidic.

> *"I was surprised how much I liked drinking the lemon juice in water each morning. To me, it just feels clean. I just felt healthier right away."*
>
> *Karla, 49 years old*

Even though it seems counterintuitive, lemon juice, which is acidic outside the body, actually becomes alkaline inside the body after it metabolizes. This happens once its minerals are dissociated in the bloodstream. It has to do with the low sugar content of lemons. If you squeeze an orange into a glass of water and drink it, it would become acidic in the body, because the sugar content of the orange would "outweigh" the alkalinizing effect of the other minerals. So, a lemon becomes alkaline in the body. Try it and see what you think. Acidity affects your gut bacteria, as well. (You didn't think your gut was immune from that, did you?) The fermentation of food in your gut is what controls the acidity level.

> *"Interestingly, I had one evening when I scarfed down a bunch of cookies. The next morning I felt a urinary tract infection coming on. I drank my lemon water and followed the plan, and it went away!"*
>
> *Susie, 51 years old*

Q: Why the smoothie for breakfast?

A: The smoothie starts the day with the nutrient-rich fruits and fiber that get the body going in a good direction. To simplify your morning routine, try combining your fruit and yogurt into a delicious smoothie in place of your normal breakfast. A 16 oz. smoothie with the whole fruit, protein and healthy fat is plenty to keep you going all morning. Another option could be to divide the smoothie recipe below into two glasses for you and another family member. If you choose the smaller smoothie, you can add it to your regular breakfast routine.

Smoothie Template

Create your own smoothie using these ingredients. Combine in a high-speed blender or smoothie blender. If you prefer a thicker smoothie, add larger quantities of frozen ingredients, use frozen bananas instead of fresh or add a couple of ice cubes

Start with one cup of one or a combination of these:
Frozen blueberries
Frozen cherries
Frozen mixed berry blend

Add ¼ cup of one of the following for creaminess factor:
Fresh bananas (for thinner smoothies)
Frozen bananas (for thicker, colder smoothies)
Frozen mango chunks

For protein and healthy fats, add 1 Tbsp. of ONE of the following:
Almond butter
Peanut butter
Coconut Oil
Your favorite protein powder
Walnuts
Cashews

Optional, add ¼ cup of ONE of these for Probiotic Boost:
Greek yogurt

Kefir

Fruit flavored organic yogurt

Soy, almond or coconut yogurt

Optional, add ONE (1 tsp.) for a dash for flavor:

Powdered Ginger

Cinnamon

Cocoa powder

Feeling adventurous? Choose one and add ¼ cup:

Fresh Spinach

Soaked whole oats

Fill to 16 oz. mark on blender with:

Unsweetened Almond milk (vanilla or original)

Water

Green tea, unsweetened and cooled

Blend thoroughly, pour into a 16 oz. glass and enjoy.

Tip: When you have bananas on the counter that are getting too ripe, peel them and break them into chunks, place them in a gallon zipper bag in the freezer. Pull out one chunk at a time, as needed.

Q: Why organic yogurt and what is kefir?

A: A good quality organic yogurt usually has more live and active cultures than many popular brands. In addition, the organic brands usually have less sugar and no fake colors. The goal is good live and active cultures, without lots of added stuff – so read the label, find a good quality brand you like, flavored is fine. A good one to try is Stonyfield Farms™. Organic yogurt may be more expensive than conventional, but you only need ¼ cup a day. Because I recommend a very small serving size, any container of yogurt will last several days. Another option is kefir. Kefir is a fermented milk drink, with a flavor similar to yogurt that usually contains more types of live and active cultures than organic yogurt. Lifeway is a popular kefir brand containing 12 live and active cultures and it is available at most grocery stores in the dairy section. It comes in organic as well as non-organic – using milk from cows not treated with pesticides, antibiotics or synthetic growth hormones or GMO feed. Again, ¼ cup each day is all you need to get ongoing digestive benefits from the live and active cultures.

> *"I hope to keep doing this! I discovered that I like yogurt… I didn't think I did."*   *Susie, 51 years old*

Q: What if I don't eat dairy?

A: Many people have dairy allergies or sensitivities. There are good non-dairy yogurts available. Try So Delicious™ coconut milk yogurt – it's organic and contains 6 live and active cultures. Other options include Silk™ soy yogurt that is not organic but the soybeans are non-GMO. Almond Dream™ almond milk yogurt is also a good choice. It is not organic but it contains 7 live and active cultures. There are many alternatives to dairy milk now, including soy, almond, coconut, hemp and rice milks. You may find you like the taste of one of these better than dairy.

Q: Which probiotic capsule should I take?

A: You will need to go to a drugstore or health food store to purchase the probiotic supplement or you can purchase it online.

Many people find it confusing to purchase probiotics, as there are many different strain combinations and various numbers on the package. Here are a few tips: You want your probiotics to be alive in order to be helpful in your digestive tract. To accomplish this, some are refrigerated and they now have effective ways of packaging self-stable probiotics, so that they stay alive. Look for a "Best Before" date or a "Guaranteed Until" date to assure you are purchasing a fresh product. First choose the *potency*. The giant number prominently displayed on the package indicates potency. Look for one that has between 1 billion and 15 billion live cultures per capsule. That is a standard potency for regular daily use. (You may see some with 30, 50 or even 100 billion live cultures per capsule. This is the "extra strength" version. This type would be great to take for a shorter duration, for example, during and after a round of antibiotics, or when you have seriously depleted your gut bacteria. The high potency type will usually be more expensive.) Choose a probiotic supplement with several *strains* of cultures; aim for 6 or 7 strains. (Some will have only one single strain such as an acidophilus supplement – don't get that type). Then there are the names of strains - full names include genus, species and strain, for example, Lactobacillus acidophilus 123SAG. Finally, most probiotic supplements will combine strains that work together in harmony and they will categorize them according to their benefits, for example, Colon Care or Women's Health. Your microbiome may need more support in one area or another. If you are a woman who tends to get yeast infections, for example, you may want to choose Women's Health. For the purposes of the 21-Day Plan, it is best to choose one for general digestive or colon health. One good quality brand that has a shelf-stable line is Renew Life™ Ultimate Flora™. This brand is widely available at drugstores, health food stores and online. Another good brand is Probiotic Pearls™ (from

Enzymatic Therapy brand). The shelf stable brands are available for $14 – $30 for a one-month supply. Usually the health food store will have several brands that are refrigerated. These are generally more expensive ($30 – $50 for a one-month supply) and usually have a guarantee of potency.

Visit my website for more information on purchasing the right probiotic supplement for your needs.

Q: Which magnesium citrate supplement should I take?

A: Magnesium citrate supplements (taken orally) are safe for most people to take on a daily basis. An exception to this would be those in kidney failure. I highly recommend a brand called Natural Calm™ that is a powdered magnesium citrate you stir into water. Take it at bedtime as it helps to calm the effects of stress and promotes a good night's sleep. It can be purchased online at www.naturalvitality.com or at the discount site www.vitacost.com. It is also available at your local health food store. The 8 oz. jar will be plenty for the 21-Day Plan. Depending on where you purchase it, it can run $13.79 – $24. There is an RDA (Recommended Daily Allowance) of magnesium that varies per age group. Below is a chart for the RDA for the different age groups.

Age (years)	Male (mg/day)	Female (mg/day)	Pregnancy (mg/day)	Lactation (mg/day)
1-3	80	80	N/A	N/A
4-8	130	130	N/A	N/A
9-13	240	240	N/A	N/A
14-18	410	360	400	360
19-30	400	310	350	310
31+	420	320	360	320

If you already take a Calcium or multivitamin supplement, you may already be taking some magnesium. Check the label. Many supplements contain a small amount of magnesium. You will want to determine how much magnesium you are currently taking, and then use the chart to calculate how much additional magnesium citrate to add to get the RDA.

For instance, if you are an adult female that is 31 years or older, your RDA is 320 mg per day.

You can properly dose yourself by comparing how much magnesium you are already getting from your other cal/mag (calcium/magnesium) supplement and then taking the difference in milligrams of the Natural Calm™. For example, if your current cal/mag supplement gives you 250 mg of magnesium, then you only need to take 60 mg of Natural Calm™. To make it easier, 1/3 teaspoon of Natural Calm™ is 80 mg. ¼ teaspoon should be more accurate for 60 mg's.

Not everyone is the same when it comes to how much magnesium they should take. Some people require more than the RDA, while others less. The good thing about magnesium is that if you take too much, your kidneys will purge the excess to your bowels and cause a loose stool. If this happens, then you know you are taking more than your body needs. Just reduce the amount until you find the right dose that works for you. *Many people prefer to start with a small dose – about ½ teaspoon, or 120 mg. Work your way up to a larger dose over several days.*

If you prefer a capsule, look for magnesium citrate capsule, rather than the plain magnesium. Take the RDA dose for your gender and age. Take it with a 4 oz. glass of water.

Ione, 72 years old, reported that her leg/foot cramps were a 7 (moderately severe) on a scale of 1 to 10 before she started. The magnesium citrate helped her tremendously and at the end of the 21-Day Plan she reported that her leg/foot cramps were a 2 (mild) on a scale of 1 to 10).

Q: What if I have trouble remembering to do the actions?

A: You will have better results if you do the actions listed for each day. Tips to help you remember: Complete the tracking chart each day. This can help remind you as you check off the actions. For many people, a visual cue helps remind them of what they need to do. Place a 12 oz. cup, a spoon and the magnesium citrate next to your bathroom sink. Take the supplement at bedtime mixed with 4 oz. water. Another tip to remember new habits is to tie them to something you already do automatically. For example, plan your exercise at the same time everyday, before or after something you do anyway. If you always eat lunch at work around 12:00, plan your 10-minute walk right after you eat.

Q: What about exercise?

A: Our bodies are meant to move. Movement helps with digestion as well as many other important functions in your body. If you are already exercising regularly, that's great. Keep doing what you are doing. If you have not been exercising, then a short walk will be a good way to start to introduce movement, which will help with digestion and your energy level. Here's how to start a regular, daily walking habit. Choose a time when you have 10 minutes. Dress appropriately for the weather. Take a watch or phone with you. Look at the time. Walk out your door. Keep walking at a pace that is comfortable for you. In five minutes, turn around and walk back home. Repeat tomorrow. You just started an exercise routine. Wasn't that simple?

Q: Which green tea should I drink?

A: I suggest unsweetened green tea, made fresh. It's easy to make your own mug of green tea. It takes only 5 minutes. You will need a mug, hot water and one or two green tea bags. I like my tea strong, so simply putting in two tea bags when steeping, provides a stronger flavor (and more anti-oxidants.) Heat the water in a teakettle. Pour the hot water over the tea bag(s) and let sit for approximately 3 minutes to steep. Remove tea bag and enjoy. You can drink the tea either hot or iced. There are many delicious green teas and green tea blends available today in your grocery store tea aisle. You will find a wide variety of boxed tea bags. Most containers have 18 – 24 tea bags and they range in price from $2.50 – $6. Bigelow, Lipton, Stash and Salada all have green teas available in the grocery store aisle. There are also some specialty brands with excellent green tea blends such as Tazo, Harney and Sons and The Republic of Tea. If you haven't tried green tea before, I recommend choosing a green tea/fruit flavor blend, such as green tea with peach blend. If you are more of an herb person, find a green tea blended with peppermint or ginger. Those herbs are also great for digestion. And if you are out and about, Starbucks and other coffee/tea shops offer several green teas, which they can make either hot or iced. *Again, remember; ask for unsweetened green tea, made fresh.* Beware of many bottled green tea drinks or green tea smoothies that may be made with as much added sugar as a soda.

> *"I do indeed feel like I sleep better, move my bowels more regularly and have more energy. I also think I am more even tempered."*
>
> *Amanda, 62 year old*

Q: How much water should I drink?

A: One key to improving digestion is getting enough water so all your systems for removing toxins and absorbing nutrients are able to be fully functioning. We have heard that we should drink 8 glasses of water a day. Most of us do not drink that much. Many people are chronically dehydrated, making it difficult for the digestion to work its best. Rather than having you measure and count glasses of water throughout the day, the 21-Day Plan builds in several extra glasses of water as you are taking supplements. The plan suggests one 12 oz. glass with lemon juice when you first wake up. Then another 12 oz. glass is taken with your probiotic supplement and a small glass (4 oz. suggested) is taken at bedtime with your magnesium citrate. In addition to the water, one mug of green tea is recommended each day. By week three that adds up to 28 oz. of water, plus one mug of green tea per day, so roughly 38 oz. that you are adding to whatever you normally drink. You do not need to stop drinking your favorite beverages – just *add in* the extra glasses of water and mug of green tea. Many people are concerned about water quality and water filtering. Those are important considerations; however, to keep the 21-Day Plan as simple and easy to implement as possible, I recommend drinking whatever water you have normally been consuming. (Note: coffee, soda and other caffeinated, sweetened or artificially sweetened beverages are not beneficial to your digestion. Water is preferred. Green tea provides many anti-oxidants and is anti-inflammatory and therefore, is counted in the beneficial category for the purposes of this plan.)

Section Two:

After Completing the 21 Day Plan

Please take some time to fill out the symptom checklist and the final questionnaire. This will help you become aware of the changes that you have experienced.

	None	Moderate	Severe
Respiratory issues	1	5	10
Known environmental allergies	1	5	10
Skin Issues	1	5	10
Itchy eyes/watery eyes	1	5	10
Known food allergies	1	5	10
Muscle weakness	1	5	10
Arthritis pain/joint pain	1	5	10
Muscle pain	1	5	10
General aches and pains	1	5	10
Leg cramps/foot cramps	1	5	10
Headaches/migraines	1	5	10
Low energy level/fatigue	1	5	10

	None	Moderate	Severe
Irritable/mood swings	1	5	10
Insomnia/poor sleep quality	1	5	10
Not waking up rested	1	5	10
Constipation	1	5	10
Diarrhea/loose stools	1	5	10
Gas	1	5	10
Belching	1	5	10
"Rock in stomach" feeling	1	5	10
Indigestion/Heartburn/Reflux	1	5	10
Bad Breath	1	5	10

	Mild	Moderate	Severe
Overweight	1	5	10
Underweight	1	5	10

Other symptoms (please list):

What changes were most noticeable to you after completing the 21-Day Plan?

Overall, (The 21-Day Plan) was clearly laid out, and I could treat it like a daily checklist which made it pretty straightforward to do everything."

-Sarah, 33 years old

In your own words, describe how you feel after completing the 21-Day Plan.

21-Day Plan Tracking Chart

WEEK 1

	Veggies	Movement	Mag. Citrate	Green Tea	Probiotic	Fruit	Smoothie	Yogurt	Lemon Juice
Day 1									
Day 2									
Day 3									
Day 4									
Day 5									
Day 6									
Day 7									

WEEK 2

	Day 8	Day 9	Day 10	Day 11	Day 12	Day 13	Day 14
Lemon Juice							
Yogurt							
Smoothie							
Fruit							
Probiotic							
Green Tea							
Mag. Citrate							
Movement							
Veggies							

WEEK 3

	Veggies	Movement	Mag. Citrate	Green Tea	Probiotic	Fruit	Smoothie	Yogurt	Lemon Juice
Day 15									
Day 16									
Day 17									
Day 18									
Day 19									
Day 20									
Day 21									

8| Check Your I.D. (Inner Doctor)

1) Ask 2) Listen 3) Take Action

A holistic approach to healing the gut involves listening to the signals from your body. Many of us have some habits, some traditions, or some routines that are not serving us well when it comes to our gut health. What if we don't know what they are? A good approach is to begin to listen to your I.D. Remember? Your Inner Doctor? First, take the time to become aware:

1) Ask

Ask yourself "Will I feel good later if I do/eat/drink this now?" or "Will this food/drink/whatever help me feel my best?"

By making choices based on what your body tells you, you can heal your digestive system and give your body the nutrition it is asking for. If you think about it, you can probably make a list off the top of your head of foods that "don't agree" with you. Most people have some foods that cause them some type of digestive discomfort after eating them.

2) Listen

Listen to what your body is telling you. Write down: "What are the foods that I know cause me digestive discomfort?"

Is that the time to pop an antacid? No. From a holistic approach, the antacid is simply a way to cover up the signals your body is sending.

The signals such as acid reflux, belching, bloating, intestinal cramping, and gas are good signs that you should avoid the offending foods or at least reduce how often you have them. Those are signals that your digestive system is having a hard time digesting that food. It can sometimes be a particular combination of foods that causes the distress. It may be helpful to keep a food journal or list of offending foods.

> *"I think everyone is going to have something that may not work for them, and that's OK"*   *Rose, 39 years old*

Each person is different. We have different taste buds, different body compositions, different genetics, different activity levels, different blood types, and different cultural traditions. There is no one diet that is perfect for everyone. Don't eat foods that cause you digestive distress just because you think they are "healthy." Check your I.D. – and eat what helps *you* feel *your* physical best.

You will have unique responses to the actions that are suggested in this book. One person may find that lemon juice "disagrees" with them. That's fine. Leave out the lemon juice and drink a large glass of water in the morning instead. Or maybe you find that the dairy yogurt and kefir are too much for your body. If you feel any intestinal distress after eating the yogurt, for example, then you may want to try one of the suggested non-dairy yogurts. Or skip the yogurt altogether and take the probiotic capsule instead. Your body has many unique processes going on every day. It may take a little while to "tweak" the actions suggested in this book to fit your body and your life. Perhaps it is a matter of timing. Perhaps you have a great morning routine in place and it is easy to remember to take supplements in the morning, but by evening you are feeling rushed and tired and you forget. You have the best of intentions at bedtime to take your magnesium citrate, but it just never happens. Fine. Take it in the morning when it works best for you.

> *"I enjoyed being more conscientious about what I eat and drink and tracking my digestion which I had taken for granted. It was an easy plan to follow and I liked the principle of adding, not subtracting 'foods' (although it made me more aware of things I should not eat and drink and helped me stay away from those items, sometimes)."*
>
> *Amanda, 62 years old*

Always keep in mind your current set of health concerns and use common sense as you are making changes to your diet and lifestyle. For example, if you have diverticulitis and you know that certain foods trigger a flare up, then avoid those foods. If your doctor has told you to limit large amounts of leafy greens due to a possible reaction with a medication you are taking, then, obviously, you would want follow your doctor's advice.

Do you need more support in your journey? Take a moment to jot down any actions you think of that you may need to take to further improve your overall health:

Now set a date (a deadline) for each item listed above to encourage yourself to take action on the important task of addressing your health issues.

3) Take Action

Make Healthy Choices

We asked. We listened. Now it is time to take action. Take a look at how you choose your food every day. Every day we get the opportunity to make choices about what we put into our digestive system. If you are at a restaurant, do you choose what to order based on what sounds good? Or what you always get? Or what the special is that day? At the grocery store, do you choose what to buy based on what is on sale or what is convenient or what is advertised? Many of us choose just out of habit. I would encourage you to start checking in with your body – have a new partner in the equation: your Inner Doctor. Start to ask yourself: What would be most nourishing? What nutrients can I give myself today? If it's true, "you are what you eat," then what do you want to be today? Ask yourself "what does my body need today to thrive?"

> *"Three months after the 21-Day Plan I have added several of the suggestions to my regular routine. The yogurt and green tea were already part of my routine, and that hasn't changed. The probiotic supplement was new, and I've kept that up. I've been trying to be more serious about regular exercise too. When I do these things faithfully, they make a difference."*
>
> *- Sarah, 33 year old woman*

We are in charge of the care and feeding of this miraculous, living organism. What are the best ingredients we can give it? Think home cooked foods. Think soothing foods. Think wholesome foods. Think real, whole fruits and vegetables, close to their natural state. If you can find organic or non-GMO foods, great! If you have a farmers market near you, shop there for fresh fruits and vegetables. Many farmers markets have meat, eggs and other animal products available as well. Stay away from prepared and processed foods as much as possible.

Choose meals that have veggies and fruits built in, such as entrée size salads, vegetable soups or vegetable-packed casseroles. Add extra veggies at the salad bar. Add grilled veggies to your burrito. Add lettuce, tomato, pickles and onion to your burger. Add fruit to your breakfast. Be unconventional – add veggies to your breakfast. Instead of a low nutrient snack like crackers, choose nuts or a spoonful of nut butter or a piece of fruit or veggies and hummus. These are all great ways to add nutrients and natural fiber to your diet.

The best food you can give your body is food that makes your body feel good and gives you the energy to do the things you love to do. And, of course, food is a great pleasure of life. So we want food to taste delicious.

> *"Making raw veggies a priority EVERY day felt great and helped control my typical sugar cravings"*   *Susie, 51 years old*

There are several generalities about foods that can help most people improve their digestion and increase their energy and mood. Remember the Native American tale? Feed the good wolf. Limit the bad guys and increase the good guys.

The Bad Guys

Processed Foods, Preservatives and Additives

Processed foods, manufactured foods, junk foods all zap your energy. Their purpose is to be convenient, addictive, fast and have a long shelf life. If you want more energy, you need to be adding in foods each day that contain energy – not dead, processed junk. Eat food that is real. Eat foods that are close to their natural state. Choose a banana over a banana nut muffin. Choose a bowl of fresh berries over a strawberry fruit roll-up. Choose steamed fresh broccoli over a frozen potpie. Choose whole chicken breasts over fried chicken strips. Choose cherries for dessert over cherry cheesecake.

Gluten

What about gluten? There is a lot of talk about gluten these days. Gluten is a protein that occurs naturally in certain grains. Gluten is found primarily in wheat, but also rye and barley, farro and spelt. Other grains such as oats are often processed in plants that process wheat, so are not strictly gluten-free, unless it is indicated on the package.

Why is gluten a problem? It is estimated that about 1 in 100 people in the U.S. have celiac disease. Celiac disease is an inherited, chronic inflammatory autoimmune disorder, which is diagnosed by a blood test from your doctor. A person with celiac disease has a reaction to gluten that causes the digestive system to attack itself, destroying the lining of the small intestine. For those with celiac disease, careful attention to adopt a gluten-free diet is critical. Many other people find they are simply sensitive to gluten and they feel better and experience fewer symptoms when they avoid it.

However, even if you do not have gluten sensitivity or celiac disease, gluten and wheat may not be doing you any favors. Most of us are getting a very large dose of processed wheat flour every day. It's in our cereal, our pancakes and waffles, our muffins, our toast, our snack bars, our sandwich, our pizza, our bread, our tortillas, our cake, our cookies and our crackers. It's also in smaller quantities in breaded coatings on meats, meat patties, sausages and fries, in snack foods, and hidden in lots of soups and sauces. It can also be found in flavorings and colorings. Regardless of whether you have gluten sensitivity, the wheat flour in these large doses every day is not nourishing our bodies very well. Most wheat products, especially the non-whole-grain wheat products are low in micronutrients and they are not giving our cells the nourishment they need. They fill us up with calories but do not nourish our bodies. I am not suggesting switching to all gluten-free breads and cookies and cakes, but rather, opting for foods that provide more nourishment by including more veggies and fruits and proteins and fats. The recipes included in this book are naturally low in gluten/wheat flour. Cutting back on this source of empty calories makes room for more nutritious foods, even if you do not choose to eliminate wheat altogether.

Dairy

A large percentage of adults (estimated at 30 million adults in the U.S.) are lactose intolerant. That means that the small intestine does not make enough of the enzyme lactase to digest the lactose in the dairy products you ingest. This can cause intestinal distress shortly after eating dairy. This will typically show up as bloating, cramps, diarrhea, gas, or nausea 20 minutes to two hours after consuming dairy. If you want to try going dairy-free, there are plenty of delicious dairy substitutes to help you transition away from milk, butter, cheese and ice cream. Most grocery store refrigerated sections now sell dairy-free, plant-based products. Try replacing your carton of milk with almond milk such as Almond Dream. Substitute Earth Balance margarine for butter. Daiya™ is a good non-dairy cheese product that comes in several varieties. And in your grocery store freezer section there are several very tasty non-dairy ice creams these days. Try Rice Dream™, Tofutti™, NadaMoo™ or one of many delicious brands of sorbet (not sherbet which contains dairy).

> *"Dairy yogurt caused congestion so I switched to coconut milk yogurt which agreed with me."*   *Ione, 72 years old*

Yogurt and kefir (yogurt drink) are recommended in the 21- Day Plan because of the live and active cultures that are so good for your gut. Many people who have trouble digesting milk are able to digest yogurt and kefir made from cow's milk. If you want to go completely dairy-free, there are several good non-dairy yogurts and kefirs that contain live and active cultures. These include Silk, Coconut Dream, and Whole Soy and more. Also keep in mind, many people can digest goat cheese or goat milk more easily than cow milk. For this reason, goat cheese has been included in a few recipes in small quantities for some creamy flavor and richness.

Red Meat

Many people enjoy eating red meat such as pork, beef, ham, and sausage, but if you are having constipation or sluggish digestion, it may benefit you to reduce your red meat consumption. It takes longer for red meat to work its way through the digestive system than fish, chicken, eggs, etc.

Sugar and Sugar Substitutes

The World Health Organization has recommended that adults limit their sugar intake to 6 teaspoons or 25 grams per day. The American Heart Association recommends no more than 9.5 teaspoons per day. The average American adult consumes 22 teaspoons of sugar per day (Suez 2014). If you have kids, it will probably not surprise you that kids eat more sugar than adults. The average American child consumes 32 teaspoons per day. One can of soda often contains up to 10 teaspoons or 40 grams of sugar. Excessive sugar consumption leads to insulin resistance, cravings and can contribute to the increase in diabetes and other health issues. Sugar substitutes don't fare much better. They are hard on the digestion and they can contribute to cravings.

A recent study suggests that artificial sweeteners cause spikes in blood sugar via an interaction with the gut bacteria (Suez 2014). After showing the connection in mice, a small trial in people caused insulin resistance in some of the subjects.

Some sugar substitutes such as sorbitol and xylitol can cause bloating and diarrhea. Sugar and sugar substitutes are bad news, and your gut will be better off without them.

Coffee

I know, I know. You are hooked on coffee. I love it, too. My husband is an espresso connoisseur and makes us custom espresso drinks. It's hard to give up coffee! But if you suffer from digestive distress and you are wondering why, you may not need to look any farther than your morning cup of coffee. The increase in stomach acid can cause acid reflux. The caffeine itself can cause loose stools or diarrhea. Both regular and decaf coffee causes inflammation in the body (Zampelas 2004).

Our bodies change over time. Just because you used to be able to drink 6 cups of coffee and still sleep well at night doesn't mean caffeine isn't affecting you negatively now. Many people have caffeine sensitivity and they do not realize it. It may be worth a try to give up the cup o' Joe for a week or two to see if it relieves any of your symptoms. If that thought terrifies you, then chances are you are dependent on the false energy that coffee delivers. It is definitely a stimulant. Believe it or not, after a few days without coffee (and maybe some extra sleep for a while to reboot), your body will step up to the task and start naturally providing that energy. If you are worried about a caffeine headache, try one of these remedies or try a combination.

Caffeine withdrawal natural remedies:

Peppermint tea

A nap

Tiger Balm on the temples (found in pharmacies or health food stores in the muscle rub section)

Cold, damp cloth on the eyes

Drink a lot of water

Take Magnesium Citrate

Hot bath with Epsom salt

If all else fails, a dose of aspirin or ibuprofen can help through the toughest times (but try to keep it short-term, because these do irritate the gut).

The Good Guys:

Fresh Fruits and Veggies

You know the scoop. Get lots of fresh fruits and veggies. Choose a variety. Eat them raw. Eat them cooked. Eat them every day.

Lean Proteins

We need protein, but many of us are getting more than enough of this macronutrient. Did you know that broccoli is a good source of protein? Try to choose cleaner sources from organic, grass fed, pastured, or wild-caught animals. And concern yourself more with making sure you are getting enough veggies.

Bone Broth

Broth – real broth made like your grandmother made it, boiling the liquid with the bones of the animal – has been shown to have a soothing affect on gut inflammation and heal the digestive system. When you boil the bones of any animal in the water, collagen, proline, glycine and glutamine are released into the broth. These benefit the immune system. There are also minerals including calcium, phosphorus, magnesium and potassium that are released into the broth that are in an easily assimilated form for the body to use. Amino acids are released that reduce inflammation. Adding some apple cider vinegar to the water before simmering helps to draw out the minerals from the bones.

My recipe for homemade chicken rice soup made with real bone broth is in Chapter 9.

Fermented Foods

Fermented foods include kefir (yogurt drink), sauerkraut, miso soup, tempeh, fermented vegetables such as kimchi, pickles and many other sour or pickled foods. The best ones for gut health will be sold in the refrigerated section (not the shelves) of the grocery store. Or make some yourself at home.

Nuts and Seeds and Healthy Fats

These nutrient rich nuggets of goodness are bursting with all kinds of micronutrients and good fats. Think about it – a seed has everything needed to create a whole new plant. It will give a good boost to your cells, as well. Plain, raw or unsalted nuts and seeds are best. Make sure to include healthy fats such as olive oil, avocados, flax seeds, fish oils, etc.

Now, when anyone asks to see your I.D., it can be a reminder to check in with your body – see if what you are eating and drinking is providing the nourishment your body needs to thrive.

9| Move It!

"I Like to… Move It"

- The Mad Stuntman, featured in Madagascar

My daughter and I like to take our dog and go walk at the beach. She and I have to look at our schedules and since it is about a 20 minute drive to the beach, we need to plan an hour and a half to get there, walk and get back home to get on to our next scheduled activity. Sometimes we even go *before* school and work. Now this requires an early wake-up call. But guess what? The dog is ready! Even though he *was* fast asleep at 5:00 am, if we grab his leash and head to the car, he's there, wagging his tail, ready to go.

Ever wonder why your dog loves walking? Ever wonder why a kid will naturally run to the playground and start climbing all over the play structure? They don't plan these activities. They don't care what time of day it is or if they have 30 minutes free before they have to be somewhere or if they have the right gym membership or workout clothes. They are more in tune with the signals of their body. They innately know their body needs to move. Your muscles are made for moving and they need regular daily movement to stay healthy. If you just pick up the leash or drive to the playground, the dog or the kid is ready to go! They live in the moment. And in that moment, if they sense an opportunity to move, they are up to the task.

In my own journey through weight loss, exercise and gut health, there were several years when I was overweight. I had two small children. I did not exercise. I did not feel I had the time or the energy to take care of myself. I felt bad and it was getting worse, not better. I went to my doctor at age 35 and told her I was falling apart. She asked me about my stress, my family, my sleep, my diet, and my hormones. She asked if the rest of my family was over-weight – or was it just me. (It was just me). She had some good suggestions but they all seemed too difficult to try.

I knew I needed to change something, but I did not know how. All of the weight loss and exercise programs seemed too daunting. I joined a gym, but I couldn't make it through my first class. I got discouraged. Then I found a program that met me where I was. It was called *The Change Your Life Challenge*. It started with baby steps.

> **Get a pedometer.** Find ten minutes when I could leave the house. I could do that – although it seemed hard at the time. I had to wait until my husband was home to watch the baby. Bring along a stopwatch. Hook on the new pedometer. Start the stopwatch. Walk out the front door and start walking down the street. In five minutes, turn around and walk back home. At home, look at the pedometer and record how many steps I took. Repeat tomorrow. Try to increase steps taken by 5 steps each day. It was that simple.

I started walking every day. Walking every day changed my life. What would it take to inspire you to begin walking *today* if you are not currently active? The 21-Day Plan will begin to heal your gut. Once your gut starts to heal, you will have more energy. Once you have more energy, you feel more motivated to continue on the path to better health and movement is part of that path.

Your body is meant to move. All your cells need you to move to keep their cycle of repair and replacement going. Your body sends you signals. Well, guess what? You send your body signals, too. Most of your body's tissues are under a constant state of construc-tion. Your cells only live 7-10 years, on average, and many soft tissues only live a matter of days or weeks. The epithelial cells lining the gut are probably only 5 days old on average. The average age of the digestive tract itself is 15.9 years (Wade 2005).

Making new cells all the time allows our body to respond to the outside environment. It allows us to change and grow and live under changing circumstances. This is your body's way of cleaning house. So that means that every 7-10 years, you have, essentially, a whole new body! The more you move, the more you send the signals back to your cells that they better repair and step up to the task ahead. Tell them you plan to use them to do some real work. When we sit on the couch all day, we send our cells the signal that we really do not need much energy today. We send the signal that not a lot of muscle strength is going to be needed. We send the signal "Cells, conserve your resources. Don't repair anything today."

The funny thing about movement and exercise is that logically we think that we have a certain amount of energy each day and if we exercise that will use up part of our limited allotment. But it simply doesn't work that way. At first, if you have not been used to moving each day, it may indeed cause you to be tired. You may even need to make time for an extra nap or rest afterwards. But it doesn't take long and, like magic, exercising actually gives you *more* energy! I find that now, when I exercise in the morning, I am actually *more* awake, with *more* energy plus I'm in a better mood – the rest of the day. And conversely, if I get to the end of the day and I am cranky with my family, I feel down, I have low energy, inevitably I look back and think, "Oh. I forgot to exercise today." Even then, at that late hour of the day, I can turn around my mood just by grabbing the dog's leash and heading outside for a quick once-around the neighborhood. Exercise is a great natural anti-depressant!

> *"You may have to age, but you don't have to rot." — Chris Crowley,*
> *author of* Younger Next Year

You are in charge of how you choose to live each day. You can go along the path of conventional society and get more and more aches and pains and injuries as the years go by *or* you can move your body each day. Sometimes the reason we don't start something is because we are afraid of failure. Well, throw that notion out the window. It doesn't have to be perfect. Nobody is perfect. Just open up the front door and start walking.

Maybe you already have an exercise program. Maybe you go to a gym regularly or maybe you walk the dog every day. Keep that going! We are all at different points on the path of exercise. If your plan is a few days a week, try adding a day each week. Or try adding a ten-minute walk on days when you do not do any other exercise. Moving every single day is a key to sending healthy signals back to your body.

Do you enjoy stretching and yoga? Try this yoga sequence that helps to stretch and move your core, or belly area.

Yoga for Digestion Sequence

(Approximately 10 minutes)

Repeat each step 3 times, with breath. Movements should be slow and soothing. Do not force any movements. These movements are intended to stretch and twist and massage the digestive system, which is basically your core. Please do not force yourself into any position that is uncomfortable.

1) Forward Fold to Forward Bend: Standing, inhale and stretch the arms overhead, pulling the shoulders down as you stretch up tall, lifting the belly. Then exhale and fold forward from the hip hinge, bending your knees if you need to, hanging like a rag doll. Inhale back up, one vertebra at a time.

2) Side Bend: Standing tall again, inhale arms overhead, then exhale and slowly bend to the right, as if your body was pressed between two pieces of glass. Straighten up and then repeat, leaning to the left.

3) Knee Rolls: Lay down with your back on the floor. Bring the right knee into your chest. Placing your right hand on the knee, slowly roll it around in circles. Relax the right leg back onto the floor. Repeat with the left knee.

4) Spinal Twist: Still lying on your back, bring both knees to the chest with your arms wrapped around the shins. Roll gently back and forth, massaging the low back. Come back to neutral, keeping the knees held into the chest, and then slowly twist them to the right while twisting the upper body to the left, stretching the left hand out to the left, keeping the left shoulder down. Turn the head in the direction of the outstretched arm. Pull the knees back to center squeezing them to the chest, then twist the knees to the left, upper body, arm and head to the right.

5) Seated twist: Sit on the floor with a straight spine. Bend the left leg into a cross-legged position, bringing the left foot towards the right buttock. Bend right knee and cross the right foot over the left thigh, keeping the right knee facing the sky and placing the right foot towards the left buttock. Inhale and bring your right arm

behind you, placing the right hand close to the buttocks and then bring the left elbow to the outside of right knee. Exhale and twist the upper body to the right, twisting from your core, looking over your right shoulder. Inhale and exhale again, twisting to your fullest. Return to center and repeat on the opposite side, switching leg positions and twisting to the left, looking over the left shoulder.

(No need to repeat this one 3 times)

6) Cat/Cow stretches: Move onto all fours with hands under the shoulders and knees under the hips. Holding this position and keeping the shoulder girdle steady, let your belly drop toward the floor, spreading the tailbone and lifting the head and neck gently up towards the sky. Inhale. Then as you exhale, tuck the tailbone under and arch the back up to the sky like an angry cat, pressing through the hands.

7) Downward Dog to Standing: From your position on all fours, stretch your arms straight out from the shoulders and tuck your toes under to press your buttocks up to the ceiling as you straighten the legs to any degree. Move your weight off your wrists by pressing the thighbones back behind you. Look back towards your feet. Hold for a few breaths, then walk the feet up to meet the hands, hang in forward fold for a few breaths and slowly stand up straight, uncurling one vertebra at a time, letting the head and neck come up last until you are standing tall.

Smile. You have just massaged your digestive system.

10| Stress, Stress Go Away

"It's not stress that kills us, it is our reaction to it."
-Hans Selye

When I was in high school, I had an unusual part time job. I played the organ for a small church on Sundays for their worship services. Organists were hard to come by. Although I wasn't even old enough to drive, I was taking organ lessons, so that was good enough for them. I practiced and I prepared each week. Yet every Sunday morning I got very anxious before the service started. Every Sunday, I would arrive early. I knew I needed to get there early because each week I would have to spend some time in the church bathroom before the service started. That's right. I would get so nervous that I would have diarrhea every single week. That was my stress response.

It was my body's way of reacting to the stress of playing in front of a congregation full of people. I tell you this story just to demonstrate the direct connection between stress and our gut. This was completely involuntary and it was also not related to anything I ate or any flu bug I had picked up. I realized then that pursuing music in college or professionally would not be a good choice for me.

Cortisol and Adrenaline

We all have stress in our lives. We have all heard that stress is bad for us. The body has several ways of responding to stress. Some of the stresses in our lives are chronic – they are repeated and ongoing for more than 3 weeks. Some stress is acute – it's a problem today, but it probably won't be an issue in 3 weeks. The body reacts to stress with a series of hormonal changes that are known as the fight or flight response. When you perceive a threat the adrenal glands produce cortisol and adrenaline, among other things. The adrenaline causes your heart rate to increase, raises your blood pressure and gives you that "adrenaline high" or "fight or flight" boost of energy. Cortisol, "the stress hormone," increases glucose to the brain and sends out a dose of substances to repair tissues in case of any damage. Cortisol also slows down the non-essential functions. This makes sense for survival – if you are facing a life or death situation, then you don't need your body putting effort at that moment into something as basic as growth and repair of tissues. Or digestion. The extremities become cold because the body moves blood away from the arms and legs and digestive system towards the large muscle groups.

> Julie lost her husband to cancer and is now raising their two kids on her own. She uses gratitude and prayer to deal with stress in her life, *"Even in the most stressful times, we have a lot to be thankful for. I often put myself to sleep by beginning a prayer of thankfulness. I never last until the end."*

The relaxation response occurs after you sense that the danger has passed. It takes at least three minutes for the messages to your nervous system to take effect, slowing the heart rate and the breathing back to normal. The blood flow returns to normal and digestive processes can resume.

The problem is, for many of us, the stressful situation becomes a stressful day and that stressful day becomes a stressful week, etc. It seems that our fight or flight system is on overdrive. Unfortunately, chronic stress – that ongoing, day-to-day stress, causes additional changes in the body. We keep that supply of cortisol flowing on a regular basis. Our bodies naturally slow down the basic functions like digestion and tissue repair and the reproductive system. Over time the chances of developing many stress-related diseases increases. Cortisol affects people in different ways. For some people, the gut is where they notice the effects. High levels of chronic stress can cause diarrhea or ulcers and can weaken the immune system. Chronic stress and cortisol can also cause a range of other health problems including anxiety, depression, sleep problems, difficulties with memory, and weight gain.

Let's talk specifically about how stress affects our gut. Our guts do not like stress. When we are under stress, the mechanisms that control our gut partially shut down. They have more important things to do, or at least that's what they "think." And digestion? Well, when we are under stress digestion gets put on the back burner. This is bad. Why? Because often our stress load is so high every single day that we *never* really get our digestion back to fully functioning – we are in a constant state of partial "shut down." Stress with a capital "S" takes over our digestive life. And we never catch up. No wonder we have weight gain. It is critical to pay attention to our stress level and take steps to reduce the effects of stress on the body. When we manage our stress well, those wild levels of cortisol and adrenaline subside. Lower cortisol levels in the body help the digestive functions get back on track.

Lois, 69 years old, is going through treatment for breast cancer. Here is how she is dealing with stress: *"Prayer, finding something to laugh about, a nice warm bath, soothing music, petting the dog, writing thank you notes, taking everything one day at a time, not taking responsibility when it's not warranted. I'm working on all of them!"*

If we are aware of our stressful triggers, we can take steps to reduce the actual amount of stress as well as our body's reaction. Some stress is unavoidable. Our approach to it, however, can dramatically improve how our body responds. Awareness is an important first step.

> **Stress:** the body's reaction to a change that requires a physical, mental or emotional adjustment or response.
> Stress can come from any situation or thought that makes you feel frustrated, angry, nervous, or anxious.

Awareness is useful when we are trying to reduce our stress. Writing down stressors can help us develop a strategy to reduce them.

Stress Awareness

Write three things that stress you out on a regular, ongoing basis: (Chronic stress lasts more than three weeks such as a health problem or financial difficulties)

1)

2)

3)

Write three things that are acutely stressful right now: (Acute stress is very stressful today but probably will not be an issue in a few weeks, such as an upcoming deadline or a flat tire)

1)

2)

3)

Write three ways that you notice the effects of stress in your body: (each person is different, but examples might include tight shoulders, stomachache, headache, tired during the day/low energy, anger easily, feeling anxious, weight gain or weight loss)

1)

2)

3)

We can take steps to change some things that cause us stress.

Brainstorm one item from list above that you may be able to actually change. Break the idea down into small parts. For example, if you wrote "work," try to narrow it down – is it a deadline at work, work politics, too many hours, too many meetings, what? Once you determine a factor that causes the most stress, think outside the box. Is there a way to reduce or eliminate the part of the stressful trigger that bothers you the most?

One thing about my stress that I can change:

Lynn deals with the daily stress of raising two kids, her older son is on the autistic spectrum. Here's one way she lets go of stress: *"I can't pass up a super hot bath with Epsom salts with lavender essential oil drizzled in. Helps me breathe through the most difficult of times! It also reminds me when I was a small child we had tons of lavender growing in the yard....takes me back to simple times when worries were something only adults did."*

Tried and True Ways to Reduce Stress

Here is a list of many helpful ways to reduce the effects of stress on our bodies. You will notice some are included in the 21-Day Plan. Most things that we do to relax are good for reducing our stress level, in general. They bring on the relaxation response, which reduces the cortisol levels. These things are great to do every day, but especially at times when we are feeling more stressed than usual. It is important to schedule them in and make them a priority. You may notice the beneficial effects immediately

Movement

That's what your muscles are made for. Exercise of any kind every day.

Stretching

Stretch your muscles. Good, old-fashioned, slow, stretching helps to release the tension that builds up in the muscle tissue.

Yoga

Take a class locally or check out an online site such as www.yogaglo.com. Yoga was designed thousands of years ago to help maintain the health of the body. Try the 10-minute yoga sequence for digestion on page 110.

Marie went through a very difficult divorce. During the most stressful time, she had no appetite, she had chest pain from the crushing stress and she lost over 30 pounds. Looking back, she says, *"I was a mess. I was broken."* Faith had been a part of her life growing up, but now she found herself falling on her knees and putting her life and her young child's life completely in God's hands. She began a regular yoga practice, taking classes at a local fitness center. The yoga helped her regain the strength she needed to get back on her feet again. She reports, *"The yoga brought peace to the chaos. It was centering."*

Good Nutrition

Eat real, whole food. Eat real fruit and real vegetables. Eat healthy proteins like eggs, nuts, beans, chicken and fish. Eating better and cleaner is especially important when we are stressed because our bodies need good, healthy food to nourish us so we are able to deal with stressful situations. Some foods are especially bad in stressful times and add to the stress our bodies are going through. At my local acupuncture clinic they call coffee liquid stress. When you are stressed, "Just Say No" to: food or drinks with fake colors, sugary foods like desserts, candy and sugary junk food, soda/diet soda, "energy" drinks and high calorie coffee drinks, fried foods and processed foods.

Bodywork

Get massage, acupuncture or other bodywork – your muscles tighten up when you are stressed and can tighten into "knots." But you can soften up those tight muscles by getting massage or acupuncture. Professional massage therapists and acupuncturists are trained to relax the knots in your muscles and can help get rid of aches and pains in your body.

If you aren't able to get in to see your massage therapist, you can get someone in your family to give you a shoulder rub or you can massage your own tight muscles.

Hydrate

Drink more water. It's easy and free.

Meditation

Mindfulness, meditation or deep breathing exercises really work to help the body let go of the effects of stress.

Prayer

Whatever your spiritual tradition, many people find comfort in turning to a higher power in good times and in bad.

Hot Bath

Take a soothing, warm bath to melt away stress. Add a handful of bath-quality Dead Sea salts and a few drops of lavender essential oil for extra detoxing.

Cup of Tea

Sit down with a relaxing cup of tea. Tip: Trade one cup of coffee a day (liquid stress) for one cup of unsweetened green tea. Caffeine in green tea is assimilated into the body differently than coffee and does not cause the jitters that coffee can cause.

Spend time with a pet

Pet your dog or cat – studies have shown that spending time with our animals reduces the stress hormone cortisol.

Sleep

Get your 7-9 hours or maybe you can squeeze in a 10-minute power nap after work.

Hugs

Give and receive hugs from friends and family – let them know you are having a stressful time.

Music

Music that you enjoy is relaxing for your brain and lowers your stress level.

Gratitude Journal

Write down 5 things that you are thankful for today – it makes you feel better AND it takes your mind off the difficult stuff.

Heat

Heat is soothing and great for tense muscles. Try an electric heating pad on low or a microwave heat pack on your shoulders or neck.

These things only help if you do them. Taking care of yourself is important and worthwhile. Which of these stress relievers sounds good to you?

The next time I feel my stress level is high, I am going to try these things:

1)

2)

3)

4)

5)

11| Gut-Friendly Recipes

"Let food be thy medicine and medicine be thy food"
- Hippocrates

What makes these recipes good for your gut health?

These recipes are delicious *and* help incorporate more fruits and veggies, easy-to-digest proteins and healthy fats into every meal to add fiber and nutrients to your day.

- Recipes use whole foods, simply prepared without a lot of highly processed ingredients.

- Healthy fats, *not* hydrogenated oils or trans fats, help to heal and soothe your digestive tract.

- No weird chemicals – your body will recognize everything.

- Recipes are naturally low in gluten and many have gluten-free options.

- Recipes do not include large amounts of dairy. The dairy that is included in small quantities is added for flavor or creaminess, not as a main ingredient. (Exception is yogurt. Non-dairy yogurt can be substituted, if preferred.)

- Recipes are low in added sugar, instead sweetened with whole fruit. (Exception is Fruit Crisp that has added sugar, but less sugar per serving compared with many other desserts)

- Recipes do not include red meat. Recipes using chicken, eggs, fish, beans and turkey are easier on the digestion than red meat.

Many of these recipes are credited to Aviva Goldfarb of The Six O'Clock Scramble. Her website www.thescramble.com offers an online family dinner planner that helps busy people get healthy meals on the table. The Scramble gives thousands of families a ready-made, healthy and seasonal dinner plan for the week (completely customizable) including side dishes and a grocery list, sent right to your inbox or phone for just a few dollars a month. The Six O'Clock Scramble recipes are used by permission.

I want to thank my mom, Alice Johnson, for her expertise in the kitchen and her dedication to a gluten-free, dairy-free diet. She contributed several of her favorite recipes and her help was invaluable in writing this book.

Hopefully you may find a few new favorites that make your body feel great.

Breakfast Recipes

Chocolate Cherry Smoothie

Total time: 5 minutes
Serves 1

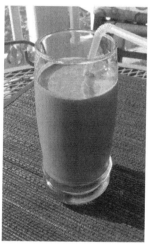

- ¾ cup frozen cherries
- ½ of a frozen banana
- 1 Tbsp. cocoa powder
- ¼ tsp. cinnamon
- ¼ cup walnut pieces
- ½ cup unsweetened vanilla almond milk or soy milk
- Water to make 16 oz.

In a blender, combine all ingredients except liquid. Pour in unsweetened vanilla almond or soymilk, then add water to the 16 oz. line on the blender jar. Blend until smooth. Makes 1 large or 2 small servings.

Nutritional Information per serving (% based upon daily values):
Calories 328, Total Fat 20.9, 32%, Saturated Fat 1.6g, 8%, Cholesterol 0mg, Sodium 93mg, 4%, Potassium 742mg, 21%, Total Carbohydrate 33.3g, 11% Dietary Fiber 8.2g, 33% Sugar 18g, Protein 10.7g

Veggie Scrambler

Total time: 15 minutes
Serves 2

- 1 cup sliced mixed peppers and onions, sold frozen as fajita vegetables
- 1 tsp. olive oil
- 4 good quality large eggs, beaten
- ¼ tsp. salt
- Pepper, to taste
- Rosemary, dried or fresh
- Salsa or diced tomato, optional

Sauté sliced peppers and onions in olive oil in a small skillet until almost tender. Add to the skillet slightly beaten eggs seasoned with salt, pepper and crushed rosemary. Cook over medium heat. As mixture cooks, lift with a spatula so that uncooked portion runs underneath. When eggs are almost set, remove skillet from heat, cover and let stand 2-3 minutes until top is set. Serve with salsa or diced tomato.

Nutritional Information per serving (% based upon daily values):
Calories 173, Total Fat 12.4, 19%, Saturated Fat 3.3g, 17%, Cholesterol 370mg, 123%, Sodium 436mg, 18%, Potassium 143mg, 4%, Total Carbohydrate 2.6g, 1% Dietary Fiber .6g, 2% Sugar 1.5g, Protein 12.3g

Yogurt Parfait

Total time: 5 minutes
Serves 1

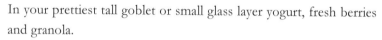

- 1 cup fruit flavored organic yogurt
- ½ c berries (fresh)
- ¼ c crunchy granola (for gluten-free granola try Bakery on Main brand)

In your prettiest tall goblet or small glass layer yogurt, fresh berries and granola.

Poached Eggs with Asparagus

Total time: 10 minutes
Serves 2

- 8-10 stalks grilled asparagus
- 2 large eggs
- salt and pepper, to taste
- sprinkle of parmesan cheese

When asparagus is in season grill extra at dinnertime and refrigerate 8-10 stalks for breakfast the next day. In small skillet or egg poacher, poach eggs. Top warmed, grilled asparagus with a poached egg and a sprinkle of Parmesan Cheese.

Oatmeal with Apple, Cinnamon and Pecans

Serves 4
Time: 15-20 minutes

- 1 cup "old-fashioned" rolled oats (gluten free, if desired)

- 2 cups water
- 1 medium apple, cored and chopped
- ½ tsp. cinnamon
- ½ cup pecans or walnuts, chopped
- Honey (optional)
- Milk or non-dairy milk (optional)

Combine 1 cup rolled oats and 2 cups water in a pot on medium heat on the stove. Bring to a simmer, stirring frequently. Turn down heat to low, if necessary. Simmer and stir until the oats reach your desired tenderness, about 3-5 minutes. Top with chopped apple, a sprinkle of cinnamon and pecans or walnuts. Flavor with a drizzle of honey, milk or non-dairy milk, if desired. Makes 4, ½ cup servings. For a healthy variation, prepare quinoa according to the package directions and serve with the same toppings as oatmeal.

Red Pepper Eggs

Total time: 10 minutes
Serves 4

- 1 Large red pepper, cored and seeded
- 4 large eggs
- spray olive oil
- salt and pepper, to taste

Slice a large red pepper crosswise into 4 ½-inch thick circles. Coat bottom of skillet with olive oil spray and preheat on low or medium heat. Lay red pepper slices in the bottom of skillet. Break an egg into each circle of red pepper. Place a cover on skillet and cook to desired degree of doneness.

Hot Rice Cereal with Almond Milk, Raisins and Walnuts

Time: about 20 minutes
Serves 4

* 1 cup Bob's Red Mill Creamy Rice Hot Cereal
* 3 cups water
* ½ tsp. salt
* ¼ cup raisins
* ½ cups walnuts
* unsweetened almond milk

Using Bob's Red Mill brand "Brown Rice Farina Creamy Rice Hot Cereal" (or other hot brown rice cereal), combine 1 cup cereal, 3 cups water and ½ tsp. salt in a pot on the stove. Bring to a boil. Reduce heat to low. Cook 5-8 minutes, stirring occasionally. Pour into 3-4 bowls, top with raisins, walnuts and unsweetened almond milk. (If you do not use all of the cooked rice cereal, pour single portions into microwavable cereal bowls, cover with plastic wrap and keep in fridge. Heat up a single bowl in the microwave tomorrow for a super-quick, gut-friendly breakfast.)

Rice Chex with Almond Milk and Sliced, Fresh Fruit

If you are a cold cereal fan, and you are trying to avoid gluten and dairy, it doesn't get any easier than a bowl of Rice Chex with unsweetened almond milk. Add sliced peaches or strawberries to the bowl or eat a piece of whole, fresh fruit on the side.

SNACK IDEAS

Apple with Peanut Butter

Enjoy an apple, cored and quartered, with peanut butter or almond butter spread on each chunk.

Veggies and Dips

Try sliced jicama, broccoli and cauliflower florets with hummus or serve baby carrots and celery sticks with ranch dip.

Steamed Green Beans with 1-Minute Peanut Sauce

Time: 15 minutes
Serves 4

- 12 oz. steam-in-bag fresh green beans
- ⅓ cup all-natural peanut butter
- Scant ½ cup water
- 1½ Tbsp. white miso paste
- Dash of soy sauce (optional)

Microwave according to package directions one 12 oz. steam-in-the-bag package of fresh green beans from the produce section. (Alternatively, wash and trim ¾ pound of fresh green beans. Boil a pot of water and boil for 3-4 minutes or until crisp tender. Drain and chill in bowl of ice water. Drain before serving.) Meanwhile, whip up Mari's 1-Minute Peanut Sauce. In a small microwavable bowl, combine peanut butter and water. Microwave on high for 1 minute. Whisk in white miso paste and whisk until mixture is blended. Adjust thickness by adding a little more water, if necessary (peanut butter consistencies vary). Add a dash of soy sauce, if desired. Cool green beans slightly, until you can pick them up with your fingers. Dip green beans in peanut sauce. Serves 4 for a snack or appetizer.

Homemade Trail Mix

About 6 ¼ cup servings

- ½ cup raw, unsalted almonds
- ½ cup raw, unsalted walnuts
- ½ cup dried cherries or raisins

For a simple mix, combine all ingredients in a zipper bag. Change it up with cashews, pumpkin seeds, dried apricots or dried apple bits. If desired, add ½ cup semi-sweet chocolate chips. Recommended serving size: ¼ cup. (Beware of many store-bought trail mixes filled with high levels of sodium, sugary coatings and processed foods.)

Half Avocado With Salsa

Time: 2 minutes

Serves 2

- 1 large, ripe avocado
- ½ cup prepared salsa

Cut a ripe avocado in half; remove the pit and spoon ¼ cup of your favorite salsa into each pit area. Spoon your snack right out of the avocado peel. One half avocado with salsa per serving.

VEGGIE SIDES

Baked Sweet Potato

Total time: 8 minutes
Serves: 1

- 1 medium sweet potato
- Olive oil

- Salt
- Cinnamon

Wash and dry a sweet potato. Pierce skin 3 times with a knife. Place sweet potato directly on microwave oven tray. Microwave on high for 5-6 minutes. (Microwave oven times vary. Give it a quick squeeze to check if it is tender.) Remove it from the microwave, slice it open, season it with a drizzle of olive oil, dash of salt and sprinkle of cinnamon. Enjoy as a quick snack or side dish. Many sweet potatoes are large enough to be cut in half or even thirds to serve several people. Add additional minutes of cooking time for larger sweet potatoes.

Baked Potato with Steamed Broccoli and Salsa

Total time: 10 minutes

Serves 1

- One medium russet baking potato
- ½ cup of broccoli florets, steamed (fresh or frozen)
- ¼ cup prepared salsa
- Olive oil

Wash and dry a russet or Yukon Gold potato. Pierce the skin with a knife. Place the potato right on the microwave tray. Microwave for 5-8 minutes, until tender. Top with a drizzle of olive oil and steamed broccoli florets and ¼ cup of your favorite salsa.

Roasted Winter Vegetables

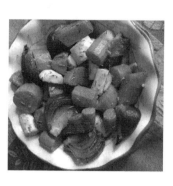

Serves 6

Total time: 45 minutes

- 2 medium sweet potatoes, peeled and cut into 1-inch chunks
- 3 carrots, peeled and cut into 1-inch chunks
- 2 medium parsnips, peeled and cut into 1-inch chunks
- 1 medium red onion, peeled and cut into 6-8 wedges
- 1 Tbsp. olive oil
- 3 cloves garlic, minced
- 1 tsp. dried thyme leaves
- 1 tsp. dried rosemary leaves
- (optional: replace thyme and rosemary with 2 tsp. Italian herb blend)
- ¼ tsp. salt
- ¼ tsp. pepper

If vegetables are wet, pat dry with paper towel and place in large bowl. Combine oil, garlic, and seasonings in a small bowl. Drizzle over vegetables and toss to coat. Place vegetables on a baking sheet with sides. Cover with foil. Bake in a 425° oven for 30 minutes. Remove foil; stir vegetables. Bake uncovered an additional 5-10 minutes or until vegetables are tender.

Quick Cooked Green Veggies

Total time: 15 minutes
Serves 4-6 as a side dish

- 1 head of Napa cabbage or Bok Choy, rinsed
- 1 Tbsp. olive oil
- ½ cup vegetable or chicken broth
- Salt (up to ¼ tsp.) and pepper, to taste

Chop one head of Napa cabbage or Bok Choy into diagonal 2-inch x ½-inch chunks. Discard the core/stem section. In a large skillet or wok (with a lid), heat 1 Tbsp. olive oil on medium high. Add vegetables and sear chunks in oil for 2-3 minutes, then lower heat to medium and add ½ cup vegetable broth. Place lid on skillet and steam until desired tenderness, 5-7 minutes. Season with salt and pepper or your favorite salt-free seasoning.

Tip: This quick-cooking method of preparing fresh vegetables works well with a wide variety of chopped vegetables. Try broccoli florets, fresh green beans, mushrooms, carrots or a combination. Adjust steaming time for firmer veggies to assure your desired tenderness.

SALADS

Classic Spinach Salad with Turkey Bacon

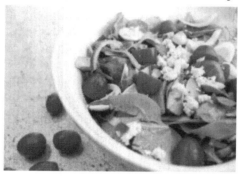

Prep+Cook Time:
20 minutes

Serves 4

- 2 eggs, hard-boiled and sliced
- 8 oz. turkey bacon
- 6 – 9 oz. baby spinach
- ¼ – ⅓ cup crumbled blue cheese, to taste, or use Gorgonzola, shredded Parmesan or feta cheese
- 1 cup sliced mushrooms, coarsely chopped
- ¼ red or yellow onion, (about ¼ cup), thinly sliced
- 1 cup cherry tomatoes, (about ½ pint), halved
- ¼ cup balsamic vinaigrette dressing, or to taste (store-bought or homemade, see below)

Hard boil the eggs, if necessary, and soak them in cold water to cool them. Peel and slice the eggs. Slice the bacon into thin strips and cook it in a large nonstick skillet over medium heat, stirring occasionally, until it is browned and crispy, 8 – 10 minutes.

In a large serving bowl, top the spinach with the eggs, cheese, mushrooms, onions and tomatoes. When the bacon is crisp, add it to the salad, top it with the dressing, and toss thoroughly. Serve it immediately.

Balsamic Vinaigrette Salad Dressing:

You can make your own easy and delicious salad dressing by whisking together ¼ cup balsamic vinegar, ⅓ cup olive oil, 1 tsp. superfine sugar (optional) and 1 tsp. minced herbs such as basil and mint. Add 1 Tbsp. Dijon mustard, if desired. Refrigerate extra dressing.

Nutritional Information per serving (% based upon daily values):
Calories 220, Total Fat 16g, 25%, Saturated Fat 4.5g, 23%, Cholesterol 155mg, 52%, Sodium 1170mg, 49%, Total Carbohydrate 4g, 1%, Dietary Fiber 5g, 20%, Sugar 2g, Protein 16g

Tuscan Tuna and White Bean Salad

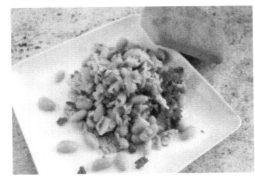

Marinate Time:
30 minutes
Prep + Cook Time:
15 minutes
Serves 4

- 30 oz. canned cannellini beans (also called white kidney beans), *drained and rinsed*
- 6.4 oz. chunk light tuna in water, *(1 pouch, drained)*
- ¼ red onion, *finely diced (about ½ cup)*
- 1 Tbsp. capers, *chopped if desired*
- 2 Tbsp. extra virgin olive oil
- 1 tsp. red wine vinegar
- ¼ lemon, *juice only, 1 Tbsp.*

continued…

- ⅛ tsp. black pepper, *or to taste*
- 10 fresh basil leaves, *chopped, or use fresh flat-leaf parsley*

In a large serving bowl, combine the beans, tuna, onions and capers.

In a small bowl, whisk together the oil, vinegar, lemon juice and pepper, pour it over the tuna mixture, and stir thoroughly to combine. Gently stir in the basil and serve it immediately or refrigerate it for up to 3 days before serving.

Nutritional Information per serving (% based upon daily values):
Calories 301, Total Fat 7.5g, 12%, Saturated Fat 1g, 5%, Cholesterol 36mg, 12%, Sodium 596mg, 25%, Total Carbohydrate 32.5g, 10.5% Dietary Fiber 10.5g, 41% Sugar 3.5g, Protein 27g

Turkey, Cranberry and Wild Rice Salad

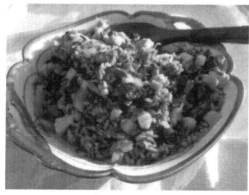

Marinate Time:
15 minutes
Prep Time:
10 minutes
Cook Time:
60 minutes
Total Time:
1 hour 25 minutes
Serves 6

- ½ cup dried cranberries, (or use raisins or pomegranate seeds) or ½ – ¾ cup cranberry sauce
- ½ cup pecans, lightly toasted and coarsely chopped
- 2 – 4 scallions, thinly sliced (¼ – ½ cup), to taste
- 2 stalks celery, sliced (about 1 cup)

- ¼ cup balsamic vinaigrette dressing, (or use equal parts olive oil and balsamic vinegar)
- 1 cup wild rice blend, such as Lundberg's
- 1 cup cooked turkey breast, chopped

Prepare the rice according to the package directions, using water or leftover chicken broth.

In a medium serving bowl, combine the turkey, celery, scallions and cranberries. When the rice is cooked, combine it with the ingredients in the bowl. Stir in the vinaigrette dressing. Refrigerate the salad for at least 15 minutes and up to 2 days. Just before serving, stir in the pecans. Season it with salt and pepper to taste.

Balsamic Vinaigrette Salad Dressing:

You can make your own easy and delicious salad dressing by whisking together ¼ cup balsamic vinegar, ⅓ cup olive oil, 1 tsp. superfine sugar (optional) and 1 tsp. minced herbs such as basil and mint. Add 1 Tbsp. Dijon mustard, if desired. Refrigerate extra dressing.

Nutritional Information per serving (% based upon daily values):
Calories 301, Total Fat 7.5g, 12%, Saturated Fat 1g, 5%, Cholesterol 36mg, 12%, Sodium 596mg, 25%, Total Carbohydrate 32.5g, 10.5% Dietary Fiber 10.5g, 41% Sugar 3.5g, Protein 27g

Spinach and Quinoa Salad with Toasted Cashews and Dried Cranberries

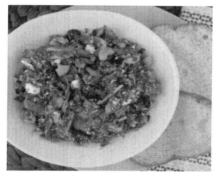

Prep + Cook Time: 25 minutes

Makes 6 servings, about 1½ cups each

- 1 cup quinoa, preferably red
- ½ – 1 lemon, juice only, ¼ cup
- ¼ cup extra virgin olive oil, (preferably something light and fruity, if you have it)
- 6 oz. baby spinach, (about 6 cups), sliced into thin strips
- 4 scallions, dark and light green parts, thinly sliced
- ¼ cup fresh dill, finely chopped, or use 1 tsp. dried
- ½ cup fresh mint leaves, chopped
- 1 cup cashews, lightly toasted, coarsely chopped, or use toasted pumpkin seeds for a nut-free alternative
- ½ cup dried cranberries
- ½ cup crumbled feta or goat cheese

Cook the quinoa according to package directions (this can be done up to 2 days in advance).

In a measuring cup or medium bowl, combine the lemon juice, oil, and dried dill, if using it (if using fresh dill, add it with the remaining salad ingredients).

In a large bowl, combine the remaining ingredients, except the cheese. Stir in the cooked quinoa and the dressing, and then gently fold in the cheese. Season it with salt and pepper to taste. Serve it immediately or refrigerate it for up to 3 days.

Nutritional Information per Serving (% based upon Daily Values):
Calories 395, Total Fat 24.5g, 37.5%, Saturated Fat 5.5g, 27.5%, Cholesterol 11mg, 3.5%, Sodium 180mg, 7.5%, Carbohydrate 38.5g, 12.5%, Dietary Fiber 5.5g, 22.5%, Sugar 9g, Protein 10g

SOUPS

Totally Homemade Chicken Soup

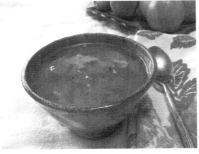

Makes 8 2-cup servings
Time: A couple of hours

I like to make this soup on a Sunday afternoon when I am working on multiple tasks around the house. It takes a couple of hours when you include the time it takes to cool and pull the chicken off the bones. The broth can also be made in a crockpot on high for 7-8 hours. This recipe makes a large batch of soup that can be eaten over several days, packed for lunches in thermoses or frozen for a busy night when you don't have time to make dinner. Herbes de Provence is an herb blend originating in France which you can find at spice shops or bulk spice stores. Your favorite herb blend will work just as well. This soup is also beneficial when your loved one is feeling under the weather – their healing time is slashed!

continued...

- 1 whole, 3.5 pound organic chicken (remove all packaging and items inside the chicken)
- 12 cups water
- 2 Tbsp. apple cider vinegar
- 1½ medium yellow onions, peeled and chopped
- ½ pound carrots, peeled and cut into chunks
- 2 stalks celery, chopped
- 1 Tbsp. sea salt (or 3 Tbsp. Better Than Bouillon No-Chicken Base or your favorite chicken bouillon)
- 1 Tbsp. Herbes de Provence (or herb blend of your choice)
- 1½ cups brown rice, uncooked

Place the whole chicken and all other ingredients except rice in a large stockpot. Bring everything to boil. (The apple cider vinegar helps to pull the nutrients from the bones of the chicken into the broth. Bone broth is soothing for your digestive system and very good for your gut health.)

Simmer on low for approximately 1 hour or longer, if time permits.

Turn off heat. Let the pot cool until chicken is cool enough to handle. Using tongs or a meat fork, lift the whole chicken onto a platter or large mixing bowl so you can work with it. Save all liquid and vegetables in the stockpot for the soup. Have another empty bowl or container nearby to place the inedible parts.

Pull apart the chicken, separating the meat from the bones and inedible parts. Discard bones and inedible parts.

Use approximately half the meat for the soup, breaking or chopping it into bite-size chunks. (I like to use 1 breast + meat off carcass and wings) You can keep the remaining meat for chicken salad or chopped chicken in a different recipe. Freeze remaining chicken meat if you will not use it within a few days. Once you have separated all chicken from the bones, you can dispose of the carcass and skin and remaining inedible parts of the chicken.

Rice:

In a separate pot or rice cooker, prepare 1½ cups of brown rice (3 cups cooked) with 4 cups water. Cook until tender.

Combine the cooked brown rice and the broth/vegetable mixture in the stockpot with the chunks of chicken meat. Heat until simmering. Try a taste and season with salt and pepper to taste.

Crockpot Split Pea Vegetable Soup

Makes 3½ Quarts of soup or 7 2-cup servings
Time: 20 minutes hands-on, 4-8 hours in crockpot

Want a hearty, warm meal to come home to in the evening? The house will smell great when you walk in if you take 10 minutes to start this soup in the morning. What? No ham? You won't miss the ham in this flavorful recipe chock full of veggies.

Place all ingredients in crockpot in the morning:

* 3 cups dry green split peas (a little more than 1 lb.)
* 8 cups water
* 2 tsp. salt
* 1 large yellow onion, chopped
* 1 tsp. crushed garlic (2 cloves, minced)
* 2 stalks celery, chopped
* 4 large carrots, peeled and chopped

Cook in crockpot on high for 4-6 hours or on low for 6-8 hours. To finish soup, add:

* 1 15 oz. can garbanzo beans, rinsed and drained

continued...

- 3 Tbsp. Balsamic vinegar
- 1 large or 2 medium tomatoes, cored and chopped
- 2 tsp. dried rosemary
- 2 tsp. dried basil
- fresh ground pepper, to taste

Taste and season with salt, if needed.

Place the lid back on the crockpot and continue to heat for 10 minutes before serving to soften tomatoes and blend the flavors.

Nutritional Information per Serving (% based upon Daily Values):
Calories 380, Total Fat 2g, 3%, Saturated Fat 0g, Cholesterol 0mg, Sodium 774mg, 32%, Carbohydrate 68.8g, 23%, Dietary Fiber 25.1g, 100%, Sugar 12.6g, Protein 24.9g

Golden Goodness Vegetable Soup

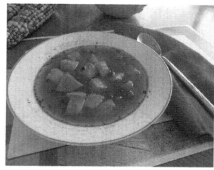

Makes 4 Quarts of soup or 8 2-cup servings Total time including cooking time: 45 minutes

- 3 Tbsp. olive oil
- 1 large yellow or white onion, peeled and chopped
- 2 cloves crushed garlic (1 tsp. jarred crushed garlic is fine)
- 5 cups peeled and cubed sweet potatoes (2 medium or 1 large sweet potato)
- 2 stalks celery, chopped
- 1 red pepper, seeded and chopped
- 1 cup frozen cut green beans

- 8 cups water
- 1 15 oz. can garbanzo beans, rinsed and drained
- 1 14.5 oz. can fire roasted diced tomatoes, with liquid
- 1 large very ripe pear, cored and diced (optional)
- 1 tsp. cinnamon
- 2 tsp. paprika
- 2 tsp. turmeric
- 2 tsp. dried basil
- Several dashes of hot sauce, more if you like some heat
- ½ cup chopped fresh parsley
- 2 Tbsp. tamari or soy sauce
- salt and freshly ground pepper, to taste

In a large stockpot, heat olive oil and add onions, garlic, red pepper, sweet potatoes, and celery. Saute for about 8 minutes. Then add green beans. Saute for an additional 4 minutes. Add water, cinnamon, paprika, turmeric, basil, hot sauce and the diced pear, if using, and bring to a boil. Turn heat to medium low to simmer for about 10 minutes until all veggies are tender.

To finish the soup, add the garbanzos, tomatoes, tamari and fresh parsley. Simmer for an additional 10 minutes until heated through and flavors have blended. Taste and season with salt and pepper, as needed.

Tips: The overripe pear is added to give the soup a natural sweetness. Ideally, the pear should almost dissolve in the soup.

This soup improves the longer you have time to let it simmer. If time permits, let it simmer an additional 20 minutes to meld the flavors.

Nutritional Information per Serving (% based upon Daily Values):
Calories 254, Total Fat 6.5g, 10%, Saturated Fat .8g, 4%, Cholesterol 0mg, Sodium 711mg, 30%, Carbohydrate 45.2g, 15%, Dietary Fiber 8.3g, 33%, Sugar 6.9g, Protein 5.8g

Roasted Sweet Potato and Apple Soup

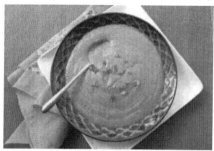

Prep Time: 20 minutes
Cook Time: 30 minutes
Total Time: 50 minutes
Makes 6 servings of 1½ cups

- 2 medium sweet potatoes, peeled and cut into medium chunks
- 1 firm apple, such as Gala or Jonagold, peeled, cored and quartered
- 1 medium yellow onion, peeled and quartered
- 2 whole cloves garlic, peeled
- 2 Tbsp. extra virgin olive oil
- ¼ tsp. salt, or to taste
- ⅛ tsp. black pepper, or to taste
- 3 – 4 cups reduced-sodium chicken or vegetable broth
- ¾ cup nonfat or low fat sour cream, for serving (optional)

Preheat the oven to 450°. Put the sweet potatoes, apples, onions and garlic in a roasting pan. Toss them with the oil and a few shakes of salt and pepper. Roast, tossing every 10 minutes, until they are soft, about 30 minutes.

Puree the vegetable/apple mixture in a blender or food processor (or in the pot using an immersion blender), adding just enough broth to cover it. Add more broth to the blender until the soup reaches the desired consistency, so it is smooth and not too thick. If you are using a blender, you will probably need to puree the soup in two batches.

Warm the soup over low heat in a stockpot until ready to serve, or refrigerate it for up to 1 day or freeze it for up to 3 months. Stir in sour cream at the table for a creamier taste, if desired.

Nutritional Information per serving (% based upon daily values):
Calories 120, Total Fat 5g, 8%, Saturated Fat 0g, 0%, Cholesterol 0mg, 0%, Sodium 310mg, 13%, Total Carbohydrate 16g, 5%, Dietary Fiber 2g, 9%, Protein 2g, Sugar 9g

FISH RECIPES

Baked Salmon with Mango Salsa

Prep + Cook Time: 40 minutes

Serves 4

Salmon:

- 4 Salmon fillets, 4 ounces each
- 1 Tbsp. olive oil
- ½ tsp. salt
- ground pepper to taste

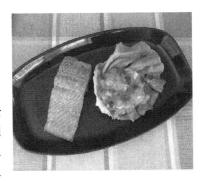

Preheat oven to 425°. Rub or brush salmon with olive oil and sprinkle with salt and pepper. Place in an oiled baking dish. Bake uncovered 15-20 minutes until fish flakes easily with a fork. Serve with chilled Mango Salsa.

Mango Salsa:

- ¼ cup fresh cilantro leaves

continued...

- 1 ripe mango, peeled and coarsely chopped (or 8 oz. frozen mango chunks, mostly thawed)
- 2 Tbsp. fresh lime juice
- ¼ of one red pepper, finely diced
- 1 green onion, sliced
- ⅛ tsp. crushed red pepper flakes

To prepare salsa, place cilantro in food processor, pulse to chop, add mango to food processor and pulse. Chop only until some mango pieces are crushed and some are still chunky. Empty contents of food processor into small bowl. Add remaining ingredients and stir to combine. Serve at once or chill until serving time. Salsa will keep overnight in refrigerator.

Nutritional Information per serving (% based upon daily values):
Calories 283, Total Fat 13g, 20%, Saturated Fat 1.9g, 9%, Cholesterol 68mg, 23%, Sodium 359mg, 15%, Total Carbohydrate 10g, 3%, Dietary Fiber 1.3g, 5%, Protein 29.8g, Sugar 8.1g

Cornmeal Crusted Fish with Black Bean Corn Salsa

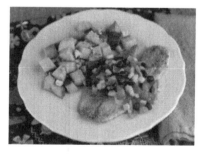

Prep + Cook Time:
30 minutes

Serves 4

- 15 oz. canned black beans, *drained and rinsed*
- 1 cup chunky salsa
- 1 cup frozen corn kernels, *or use fresh or canned*

- ⅓ cup yellow cornmeal
- 2 tsp. Old Bay seasoning
- 1 lb. tilapia, catfish, trout, or other white fish fillets
- 1 – 2 Tbsp. extra virgin olive oil

In a small saucepan, combine the beans and salsa and bring them to a boil. Add the corn and simmer it for 5 – 10 minutes, stirring occasionally, until it is heated through. Keep it warm over low heat until the fish is ready.

On a shallow plate, mix the cornmeal and Old Bay seasoning together thoroughly with a fork. Pat the fish dry with paper towels, if necessary, and dredge the fillets in the cornmeal mixture, patting on extra coating to completely cover the fish. Set the fillets aside.

Coat a large heavy skillet with nonstick cooking spray. Heat it over medium-high heat, and add 1 Tbsp. oil. When the pan is very hot, cook the fillets for 4 – 5 minutes per side without moving them, until the bottoms are lightly browned (if they overlap in one pan, use two pans or cook them in two batches). If the fillets are starting to stick to the pan, add the additional Tbsp. of oil after flipping them. If they are browning too quickly, reduce the heat.

Spoon the salsa into individual bowls or spoon it on top of the fish for serving.

Nutritional Information per serving (% based upon daily values):
Calories 350, Total Fat 14g, 22%, Sat. Fat 2.5g, 13%, Cholesterol 55mg, 18%, Sodium 830mg, 35%, Total Carb. 33g, 11%, Dietary Fiber 7g, 28%, Sugar 4g, Protein 25g

Pan-Fried Tilapia with Baby Spinach

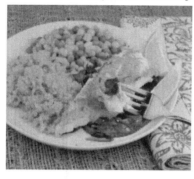

Prep + Cook Time:
10 minutes

4 Servings

- 3 Tbsp. extra virgin olive oil
- 1 tsp. minced garlic, *(1 – 2 cloves)*
- 9 – 12 oz. baby spinach
- 1½ lemons
- ¼ – ½ tsp. salt, *to taste*
- 1½ lbs. tilapia or other mild white fish fillets
- ⅛ tsp. black pepper

In a large skillet, heat 1 Tbsp. of the oil over medium heat. Add the garlic and sauté it until it is fragrant, about 30 seconds. Add the spinach, cover the pan, and cook the spinach, stirring occasionally, until it is wilted, 3-5 minutes. Uncover the pan and sprinkle the spinach with the juice of half of a lemon and season it with salt. Remove it from the heat, cover the pan, and set it aside.

In a large nonstick skillet, heat the remaining 2 Tbsp. oil over medium-high heat. Place the fillets in the pan and press them down with a spatula to ensure each fillet is completely touching the pan. Cook the fillets 2-3 minutes per side until they are lightly browned. After flipping the fish, sprinkle the fillets with the juice of another half of a lemon, and season them with salt and pepper.

Put a scoop of spinach on each dinner plate, and top it with the tilapia. Serve the dish with lemon wedges.

Nutritional Information per serving (% based upon daily values):
Calories 180, Total Fat 7g, 10%, Saturated Fat 1.5g, 7%, Cholesterol 70 mg, 23%, Sodium 85 mg, 4%, Total Carbohydrate 2g, 1%, Dietary Fiber <1g, 2%, Protein 26g, Sugar 0g

CHICKEN AND TURKEY RECIPES

Spicy Szechuan Green Beans and Ground Turkey

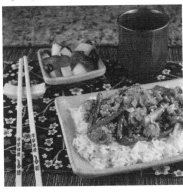

Prep + Cook Time:
25 minutes

4 Servings

- 3 Tbsp. reduced-sodium soy sauce or tamari (use wheat/ gluten-free if needed)
- 1 Tbsp. rice wine, mirin or dry sherry
- 1 tsp. brown sugar
- 1 tsp. cornstarch
- ¼ – ½ tsp. crushed red pepper flakes, *to taste (optional)*
- 1 Tbsp. vegetable or coconut oil
- 1 lb. green beans, *ends trimmed and cut in half, or use frozen*
- 1 lb. ground turkey or meatless crumble
- 2 tsp. minced garlic, *(3 – 4 cloves)*
- 1 Tbsp. fresh ginger, *peeled and minced*
- ¼ cup scallions or chives, *thinly sliced*

continued:

In a small bowl or measuring cup, whisk together the soy sauce, rice wine, brown sugar, cornstarch and red pepper flakes (optional). Set it aside.

Heat a large nonstick skillet over high heat and add the oil. When it is smoking, add the beans (if using frozen beans, defrost them first) and cook, stirring frequently, until they are shriveled and black in spots, 5 – 8 minutes. Reduce the heat if necessary to keep them from burning. Transfer the beans to a plate.

Reduce the heat to medium and add the turkey, pork or meatless crumble. Cook until no pink remains, about 5 minutes, then add the garlic and ginger, stirring until fragrant, about 1 minute. Return the beans to the pan, stir the sauce again, and add it to the pan. Cook until heated through and the sauce is thickened, about 1 minute. Stir in the scallions or chives and serve it immediately, or refrigerate it for up to 3 days, or freeze it for up to 3 months.

Nutritional Information per Serving (% based upon Daily Values):
Calories 244, Total Fat 11.5g, 18%, Saturated Fat 5.5g, 27%, Cholesterol 80mg, 26.5%, Sodium 557.5mg, 23%, Carbohydrate 13.5g, 4.5%, Dietary Fiber 4g, 16.5%, Sugar 3.5g, Protein 25g

Moroccan Chicken with Red Peppers and Carrots

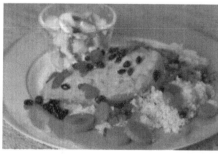

Prep + Cook Time: 30 minutes

4 Servings, about 2 cups each

- ¼ cup currants or raisins

- ¼ cup currant jelly, *or use apricot jelly or jam*
- ¼ cup white wine, *or use chicken broth*
- 2 Tbsp. reduced-sodium soy sauce (use wheat/gluten-free if needed)
- 1 tsp. curry powder
- ¼ tsp. cinnamon
- 1 Tbsp. extra virgin olive oil
- 1½ – 2 lbs. boneless, skinless chicken breasts or thighs, *cut into 1-inch pieces*
- 1 red bell pepper, *chopped*
- 2 carrots, *sliced*

In a small bowl, combine the currants or raisins, jelly, wine, soy sauce, curry and cinnamon. Set it aside.

In a large heavy skillet, heat the oil over medium heat. Cook the chicken pieces, peppers and carrots, stirring occasionally, until the chicken is fully cooked, about 8 minutes

Stir the currant mixture into the skillet and cook for about 2 more minutes or until the sauce is slightly thickened. Serve it immediately, or refrigerate it for up to 24 hours.

Nutritional Information per serving (% based upon daily values):
Calories 330, Total Fat 6g, 9%, Saturated Fat 1g, 5%, Cholesterol 100mg, 33%, Sodium 790mg, 33%, Total Carbohydrate 25g, 8%, Dietary Fiber 3g, 12%, Protein 42g, Sugar 17g

Cool Mediterranean Rice Pilaf with Chicken

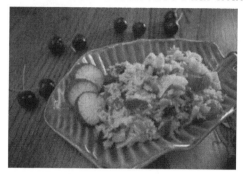

Prep + Cook Time: 25 minutes

6 Servings, about 1¾ cups each

- 2 pkgs. (6 oz. each) Near East or other brand rice pilaf mix, regular or with toasted pine nuts, or use 6 cups cooked rice for gluten-free option
- 4 stalks hearts of palm (sold in jar or can), *halved lengthwise and chopped*
- 10 sundried tomatoes, marinated in oil, *drained and chopped*
- 20 pitted kalamata olives, *chopped*
- 2 plum or Roma tomatoes, *or 1 large tomato, diced*
- 2 scallions, *all the green and most of the white parts, sliced*
- 1 cup cooked chicken breast, *diced (optional)*
- 1 cup crumbled feta cheese *(optional)*
- 2 Tbsp. extra virgin olive oil
- 1 – 2 Tbsp. red wine vinegar, *to taste*

Prepare the rice pilaf according to the package directions, using the spice pack and omitting the oil or butter.

While the rice is cooking, combine the hearts of palm, sundried tomatoes, olives, fresh tomatoes and scallions in a large bowl.

When the rice pilaf is finished cooking, fluff the rice, remove it from the heat, and let it cool for several minutes before adding it to the vegetables in the bowl. Add the chicken and/or cheese (optional), oil and vinegar and toss.

Serve the salad warm or at room temperature. You can refrigerate it for up to 2 days before serving.

Nutritional Information per serving (with chicken, not feta) (% based upon daily values): Calories 340, Total Fat 11g, 17%, Saturated Fat 1.5g, 8%, Cholesterol 20mg, 7%, Sodium 1160mg, 48%, Total Carbohydrate 49g, 16%, Dietary Fiber 2g, 8%, Protein 13g, Sugar <1g

DESSERTS

Yogurt with Fruit

If you want something sweet after dinner, try a bowl of peach yogurt with a whole peach sliced up on top. Or spoon up strawberry banana yogurt with a banana sliced on top.

Summertime Fruit Dessert

Fruit:

- ½ of a large watermelon, seeded and cut into bite-sized chunks
- 2 cups fresh blueberries
- 2 cups frozen mango chunks (or 2 mangoes, peeled and cut into bite-sized chunks)

Dressing:

- Zest of 1 lime
- 1 Tbsp. fresh lime juice
- 3 Tbsp. orange juice
- 8 fresh mint leaves, minced
- 1½ tsp. sugar or honey

Stir lime zest, juices, mint and sugar in a large mixing bowl until sugar is dissolved. Add fruit and toss gently in the dressing. Chill several hours or overnight.

Blueberry Crisp (Or Cherry Crisp)

Serves 8

Thaw time: hours

Prep time: 10 minutes

Baking time: 45 minutes

I buy the large 3 or 4 pound bags of frozen blueberries or cherries. They can be found in the wholesale clubs if you do not have the large size bags in your local grocery store.

To thaw fruit, measure out the amount you need, about 3 pounds, and place in an 8 inch round or 9 inch square baking dish and set it out on the counter for several hours to thaw.

In 8 inch round or 9-inch square baking dish, place the following:

Fruit base:

*   9 cups of thawed blueberries or cherries, pitted (a 3 lb. bag, frozen)
*   2 Tbsp. sugar, sprinkled over the top
*   1½ Tbsp. minute tapioca, sprinkled over the top
*   ½ tsp. almond extract

Gently stir to blend in baking dish. Let stand while you prepare the topping.

Crisp Topping:

Place ingredients in a small bowl or food processor:

*   6 Tbsp. unsalted butter
*   ½ cup light brown sugar
*   ½ cup unbleached white flour (use rice flour for gluten-free option)
*   ½ cup rolled gluten-free oats or rolled oats (not quick oats)

- ¼ tsp. salt
- ½ tsp. nutmeg
- 2 tsp. cinnamon

Using handheld pastry blender or food processor, chop butter and combine all topping ingredients until crumbly. Carefully spread crumbly mixture over the top of the fruit mixture in the baking dish.

Bake at 375° for 40-45 minutes.

Nutritional Information per Serving (% based upon Daily Values):
Calories 253, Total Fat 9.3g, 14%, Saturated Fat 5.5g, 28%, Cholesterol 23mg, 8%, Sodium 139mg, 6%, Carbohydrate 43.6g, 15%, Dietary Fiber 4.5g, 18%, Sugar 28.2g, Protein 2.2g

Suggestions for Eating Out:

What to do when you don't have time to prepare a meal at home?

One tip is to skip the fries and drinks – that's where many of the bad-for-your-gut ingredients hide. Order water or unsweetened tea with your meal. Here are a few dining options that include some of the good guys and fewer of the bad guys:

Fast Food:

Food Court: Entrée size salad or Caesar salad with grilled chicken

Wendy's: Broccoli and Cheese Baked Potato

McDonald's or Starbucks: Oatmeal with chopped or dried fruit and nuts

Starbucks: Bistro Boxes (varying selections of fresh fruit slices, hard boiled egg or chicken or hummus, cheeses, fresh veggies, nuts or nut butter)

Culvers: Veggie Burger topped with tomato, lettuce, pickles and onions

Taco Bell: 7-layer burrito

Jimmy John's: #4 Turkey Tom or #6 Vegetarian Sandwich

Subway: Fresh Fit Choices such as Oven Roasted Chicken 6 inch sub with extra veggies or Turkey Breast 6 inch sub with extra veggies or Veggie Delite 6 inch sub with extra veggies

Fast Casual:

Panera Bread: Black Bean Soup or Garden Vegetable Soup, Greek, Classic or Caesar Salad with Chicken, choose the apple as a side

Noodles and Company: Pad Thai Noodles with tofu or chicken and ask for extra broccoli

Chipotle: Chicken Bowl with extra grilled veggies

Suggestions for a sit down restaurant:

Appetizer: Shrimp cocktail or Minestrone soup or side garden salad

Entrée: Grilled salmon or grilled chicken with side of veggies

Salad bar with a variety of veggies and oil and vinegar dressing

Entrée size salad topped with grilled chicken or salmon

12| Conclusion

"All disease begins in the gut"   *- Hippocrates*

Your body sends many signals – cries for help – when it is having trouble keeping things in balance. When we know what to listen for, we become more sensitive to the cues. Our chronic health issues are like puzzles – each person is different and the health issues seem complex and difficult to piece together. It is your job to figure out which pieces you need to make your puzzle whole again. Many of the solutions are available to us right at the grocery store or in our homes. Real, nutritious food, better sleep, more water, taking care of our gut, reducing stress and regular movement every day all help your body to feel its best.

As you try the suggestions in this book, combining them with other healthy habits you already have, take note of how your body responds. With certain changes, you may notice a big improvement in your symptoms. With others, you will not notice a big change. Sometimes you will experience a negative effect. Remember to listen to your body. Do what works *for you*. Keep that internal dialogue going. Over time, you will begin to notice long-term improvements.

> *"I now know my exact recipe for great digestion = lemon water, yogurt, green tea, movement and fruits/ vegetables…with sufficient water!"*
> *- Rose, 39 years old*

What might you notice

What might you notice when you have better digestive health?

You sleep better. Notice any subtle changes – you do not wake up as often in the night or you get back to sleep easier when you do wake up. Perhaps you fall asleep faster when you go to bed. You have more energy in the morning. You wake up refreshed, without the alarm.

Your digestion works better. This can be noticed in better elimination habits – perhaps more regular or less painful. Perhaps your appetite is more balanced or you have fewer cravings. You may notice that you have less abdominal pain or less acid reflux.

You might notice a reduction in belly fat or bloating, gas or belching.

You may notice fewer aches and pains.

You may feel more aware or more alert when you are completing important tasks.

Your mood may improve. You may notice a more positive attitude, you may feel more resilient – better able to handle a stressful situation. Or maybe your anger or irritation is not as evident.

Your immune system will be on track to fight off colds, flus and other nasty illnesses.

How will it feel in three weeks when you feel better, your digestion has improved, you are sleeping better? What will you do with the extra energy you have? What will that mean for your life? Notice the advantages.

Muscle pain and weakness can improve when our gut is working better. Ione, age 72, reported significant improvement in her pain level after completing the 21-Day Plan. Muscle weakness in her knees went from a 7 (moderately severe) to a 5 (moderate) on a scale of 1 to 10. Her neck pain went from a 5 (moderate) to a 3 (mild) on a scale of 1 to 10. And her general aches and pains went from a 3 (mild) to a 2 (almost none) on a scale of 1 to 10.

Each person's journey is different. You may find that some parts of the program work well for you but one or two parts are difficult to fit into your schedule. You may find a new love of lemon juice and water first thing in the morning. You may find one part doesn't feel right. That is all good information. Take all that you are trying and learning and tweak it to work best for you. If one part doesn't feel right, change it but keep up the other parts. Listen to your body. That is the key.

"Two months ago I did the 21-Day Plan and it has become integrated into my everyday life. I don't even think about it anymore. I do my lemon water. I do yogurt, probiotics in my smoothie. And a lot more water than I used to drink. Every day. Without fail. And I am in a much better place with my digestive tract. For sure."

- Rose, 39 years old

You now have everything you need to begin on the path to improving your digestion. You have a better understanding of your digestive system. You know much more about some of the habits that wreck our fragile systems. You know step-by-step what to do to add more fiber, water, probiotics and movement into your life.

You have information about how to make your system more alkaline to reduce inflammation in your whole body. You have recipes and tools to help you as you make changes. You have more information about how to listen better to the signals your body is sending and check with your Inner Doctor.

Once you have completed the 21-Day Plan and you are feeling better, your digestion is working better and you are getting some movement in every day, you may start to ask, what now? Should I stop? Please don't. These changes are great to incorporate into your everyday habits. Look at the changes you have made. Look at how good you feel after only a short period of time. Over a longer period of time, your body responds and feels even better. That daily movement? Over time it helps build muscle, gets your heart rate up, and also helps keep depression at bay. Those fruits and veggies? The nutrients in them nourish your cells especially now that they can be more easily absorbed into your better functioning digestive system. The more sound sleep? That helps with your energy, your thinking, and your immune system and even helps regulate your appetite. Imagine what is going on inside your body when you are feeling this good. Imagine your cells and all your functions humming along at their best level.

Remember your car? We can't get a whole new body overnight the way we can buy a new car. But by implementing the 21-Day Plan you can give your current model an overhaul. What do you look for when buying a car? You want to make sure the car has lots of good years left in it. You want it to be reliable. You want some good features, and of course, you want it to look good. These are the same things we want for our body! It's the one and only body we get. It's time to take action. Success follows action. This is important stuff. Your health and your life depend on it. What have you got to lose? Get started today.

Acknowledgements

I would like to thank my husband, Doug, who has been supportive of this project since the start.

I would like to thank my parents, Bob and Alice Johnson, who have been my biggest fans since Day One.

I am very grateful for my editor, Bob Thorson, whose insights and gentle corrections helped this book take shape.

I thank all of you who have participated in the 21-Day Plan and who have been willing to share your experience and feedback to bring this book to life. I wish you all the best on your health journey.

I appreciate the assistance of Amanda Freymann, yoga teacher RYT200, in designing the Yoga For Digestion Sequence.

Finally, if it were not for Lindsey Smith and Joshua Rosenthal, this book would still be in my head. Thank You.

References

Alcock, Joe, Maley, Carlo C, Aktipis, C. Athena. "Is Eating Behavior Manipulated By the Gastrointestinal Microbiota? Evolutionary Pressures and Potential Mechanisms" *Bioessays* (2014). Web.

"Adult Obesity Facts." *Centers for Disease Control and Prevention.* 09 July 2014. Web.

"Antibiotic Prescribing and Use." *Center for Healthcare Research & Transformation.* Feb. 2011. Web.

"Antibiotic Use Overview." *Center for Disease Dynamics, Economics & Policy.* 2011. Web.

Blaser, Martin. "Antibiotic Overuse: Stop the Killing of Beneficial Bacteria." *Nature* 476.7361 (2011): 393-94. Web.

"Do McDonald's Burgers Contain Beef from up to 100 or Even 1000 Different Cows?" *McDonald's UK/Questions.* Dec. 2012. Web.

"Everything Added to Food in the United States (EAFUS)." *US FDA.* Nov. 2011. Web.

"Fact: You Carry Around Enough Bacteria To Fill A Large Soup Can." *Popular Science.* Sept. 2011. Web.

Fuhrman, Joel M.D. *Disease-proof Your Child: Feeding Kids Right.* New York: St. Martin's, 2005. Print.

Galland, Leo, M.D. "LEAKY GUT SYNDROMES: BREAKING THE VICIOUS CYCLE." *Foundation for Integrated Medicine.* Renaissance Workshops Ltd., 2007. Web.

Glickman, Dan. *Accelerating Progress in Obesity Prevention: Solving the Weight of the Nation.* Washington, DC: National Academies, 2012. Print.

Grice, Elizabeth A., and Julia A. Segre. "The Skin Microbiome." *Nature Reviews Microbiology* 9.4 (2011): 244-53. Web.

Guarner, F., and J. Malagelada. "Gut Flora in Health and Disease." *The Lancet* 361.9356 (2003): 512-19. Web.

"How Many Calories Do Bacteria Consume? -." *The Naked Scientists.* 12 June 2011. Web.

Hsiao, Elaine Y., Sara W. Mcbride, et al. "Microbiota Modulate Behavioral and Physiological Abnormalities Associated with Neurodevelopmental Disorders." *Cell 155.7* (2013): 1451-463. Web.

Koeth, Robert A., Zeneng Wang, Bruce S. Levison, et. al. "Intestinal Microbiota Metabolism of L-carnitine, a Nutrient in Red Meat, Promotes Atherosclerosis." *Nature Medicine* 19.5 (2013): 576-85. Web.

Lenoir, Magalie, Fuschia Serre, Lauriane Cantin, and Serge H. Ahmed. "Intense Sweetness Surpasses Cocaine Reward." Ed. Bernhard Baune. *PLoS ONE 2.8* (2007): E698. Web.

Makarieva, A. M., V. G. Gorshkov, and B.-L. Li. "Energetics of the Smallest: Do Bacteria Breathe at the Same Rate as Whales?" *Proceedings of the Royal Society B: Biological Sciences* 272.1577 (2005): 2219-224. Web.

"McDonald's McWraps. A Nutritious Choice?" *Fooducate - Eat a Bit Better.* 27 Mar. 2013. Web.

Mesnage, R., E. Clair, S. Gress, C. Then, A. Székács, and G.-E. Séralini. "Cytotoxicity on Human Cells of Cry1Ab and Cry1Ac Bt Insecticidal Toxins Alone or with a Glyphosate-based Herbicide." *Journal of Applied Toxicology* (2012): N/a. Web.

"Most U.S. Antibiotics Go to Animal Agriculture" *Food Safety News.* Feb. 2011. Web.

Newberry, Sydne J. "Probiotics for the Prevention and Treatment of Antibiotic-Associated Diarrhea." *Jama* 307.18 (2012): 1959. Web.

"Adult Obesity Facts" *Center for Disease Control and Prevention.* Sep. 3 2014. Web.

"Obesity Update" *OECD Directorate For Employment, Labour, And Social Affairs.* 2014. Web.

"Obesity Threatens to Cut U.S. Life Expectancy, New Analysis Suggests" *NIH News.* 2005. Web.

Pendick, Daniel. "New Study Links L-Carnitine in Red Meat to Heart Disease." *Harvard Men's Health Watch.* Apr. 2013. Web.

Pollan, Michael. "Some of My Best Friends are Germs," *NYTimes Magazine.* 15 May 2013. Web.

Pollan, Michael. The Omnivore's Dilemma. New York: Penguin Books, 2007. Print.

"Preliminary Characterization of the American Gut Population." 4 July 2014. Web.

"Quick, Inexpensive and a 90 Percent Cure Rate." *Mayo Clinic: For Medical Professionals.* The Mayo Foundation for Medical Education and Research, 2014. Web.

Samsel, Anthony, and Stephanie Seneff. "Glyphosate's Suppression of Cytochrome P450 Enzymes and Amino Acid Biosynthesis by the Gut Microbiome: Pathways to Modern Diseases." *Entropy* 15.4 (2013): 1416-463. Web.

Sears, Cynthia L. "A Dynamic Partnership: Celebrating Our Gut Flora." *Anaerobe* 11 (5) (2005): 247-51. Web.

Smith, Jeffrey M. *Seeds of Deception.* Fairfield, IA: Yes, 2003. Print.

Stoller-Conrad, Jessica. "Probiotic Therapy Alleviates Autism-like Behaviors in Mice." *The California Institute of Technology.* 12 May 2013. Web.

Suez, Jotham, Tal Korem, David Zeevi, et al.. "Artificial Sweeteners Induce Glucose Intolerance by Altering the Gut Microbiota." *Nature (2014).* 17 Sept. 2014. Web. "Sugar 101" *The American Heart Association.* 24 Feb 2014. Web.

Taubes, Gary. "What Really Makes Us Fat." *The New York Times.* The New York Times, 30 June 2012. Web.

"USDA ERS - Home." Economic Research Service. *United States Department of Agriculture*, 2014. Web.

Vighi, G., F. Marcucci, L. Sensi, G. Di Cara, and F. Frati. "Allergy and the Gastrointestinal System." *Clinical & Experimental Immunology* 153 (2008): 3-6. Web.

Wade, Nicholas. "Your Body Is Younger Than You Think." The New York Times. *The New York Tim*es, 01 Aug. 2005. Web.

Warner, Melanie. *Pandora's Lunchbox: How Processed Food Took over the American Meal.* New York: Scriber, 2013. Print.

Wright, Anne L., and Richard J. Schanler. "The Resurgence of Breastfeeding at the End of the Second Millennium." *Journal of Nutrition* 131.2 (2001): 421S-255. Web.

Zampelas, A., D.b. Panagiotakos, C. Pitsavos, C. Chrysohoou, and C. Stefanadis. "W01.99 Associations between Coffee Consumption and Inflammatory Markers, in Healthy Individuals: The "Attica" Study." *Atherosclerosis Supplements* 5.1 (2004): 23. Web.

Recommended Resources

More Gut Guide 101 Resources:

Visit www.gutguide101.com to sign up for free tips on improving your digestion and increasing your energy. Check the website for upcoming webinars and workshops.

One-on-one health coaching and workshops available at Alive and Well Health and Wellness.

Mari Johnson Hahn is an inspirational workshop leader and speaker. Contact her to speak at your workplace or event.

Contact Mari Johnson Hahn at:
mari@gutguide101.com.

Books recommended by the author:

The Younger Next Year books by Chris Crowley et al.

"Live Strong, Fit, and Sexy – Until You're 80 and Beyond" If you want to give your fitness and lifestyle a big kick in the pants, read these books. Chris Crowley is inspiring, funny and at 80 years old, he really practices what he preaches.

The Relaxation and Stress Reduction Workbook by Martha Davis et al.

This classic workbook-style resource has been around for years but the information is just as fresh and necessary today as it ever was.

The Change Your Life Challenge by Brook Noel. Published by Sourcebooks, Chicago, IL. For more information visit www.brooknoel.com

This book and accompanying website will meet you where you are and take you to the next level whether you need help with keeping your papers organized, getting your health back on track or a system for cleaning your home.

Happy, Healthy Gut: The Natural Diet Solution to Curing IBS and Other Chronic Digestive Disorders by Jennifer Browne

Detailed information for those who want a natural approach to curing serious, digestive conditions.

It Starts With Food by Dallas and Melissa Hartwig

This book will guide you through a 30-Day elimination diet emphasizing nutrient-dense, unprocessed food and this couple does a great job of explaining why you will want to try it.

The End of Overeating by David A. Kessler

Written by the former commissioner of the FDA, this book will give you insight into how the food industry manipulates us as consumers and how to take back control.

Eat for Health by Joel Fuhrman

Convincing resource for learning more about the nutrient density of foods and how to get the most nutritious food into your diet.

The Yoga of Eating by Charles Eisenstein.

This book is a great resource for helping you discover and change your psychological relationship with food, which is just as important as practical changes in your diet.

Movies:

Fed Up   www.fedupmovie.com

Katie Couric narrates this mainstream documentary. It is a big wake-up call to us all to become aware of the huge increase in sugar consumption in the U.S and the consequences on our health and the health of our children. "Including captivating interviews with the country's leading experts, this vital information could change the way we eat forever."

Genetic Roulette: The Gamble of Our Lives

A film by bestselling author Jeffrey M. Smith, raises awareness of the dangers of GMOs. Interviews with many experts in the field and provides details of potential health consequences of genetically modified foods.

Websites:

Elimination Diet Printable One-Sheet from www.doctoroz.com.

www.mindbodygreen.com Daily articles on holistic health topics.

www.humanfoodproject.com Mapping the microbial diversity of the American gut, along with Jeff Leach's blog.

Six O Clock Scramble: www.thescramble.com

www.yogaglo.com Hundreds of yoga and meditation classes online for a monthly fee.

www.chopracentermeditation.com Online guided meditations from Deepak Chopra.

www.responsibletechnology.org Online resource for up-to-date information about GMO foods .

www.nongmoshoppingguide.com Download a free shopping guide here if you are trying to avoid genetically modified foods.

www.thefecaltransplantfoundation.org Current listing of physicians in the U.S. who are performing fecal transplants for patients with *C. Diff.* infection.

www.openbiome.org Founded in 2012, this organization collects, screens, filters and freezes fecal matter for use in fecal transplants or FMT (Fecal Microbiota Transplantation) procedures.

Apps to inspire health:

101 Revolutionary Ways to be Healthy – Daily articles on healthy lifestyle topics

Inner Balance – This app uses a hardware heart-rate ear clip and biofeedback to teach the user how to achieve a "coherent" state that reduces stress and anxiety.

Tear-out Shopping List for 21-Day Plan

Grocery Store – Week One:

____4 lemons

____Smoothie Supplies

____Organic yogurt or kefir (enough for 7 small servings)

Grocery Store – Week Two:

____Box of green tea bags or green tea/fruit blend tea bags, at least 14 bags

____4 lemons

____2 bananas

____2 apples

____2 pears

____2 servings of fresh strawberries or blueberries

____Organic yogurt or kefir (enough for 7 small servings)

Grocery Store – Week Three:

____4 lemons

____2 bananas

____2 apples

____2 pears

____2 servings of fresh strawberries or blueberries

____Organic yogurt or kefir (enough for 7 small servings)

____Broccoli or green beans or leafy greens or ingredients for small garden salads, enough for 7 large servings

____Sauerkraut or kimchi or other fermented vegetables (found in refrigerated aisle)

Health Food Store/Drugstore/Online – One shopping trip for the whole 21-Day Plan:

____ Probiotic supplement, at least 21 capsules

____ Natural Calm™ Magnesium Citrate supplement, 8 oz. jar

Index